The
DREAM BODY
PLAYBOOK

The *ONE* and *ONLY* guide you'll ever
need to transform your body *effortlessly*

Andy Xiong

DISCLAIMER

This book is for general fitness and health, geared towards the average healthy individual. This book should NEVER be used for any medical purposes, such as diagnoses, treatments, cures, preventions or interventions. Medical recommendations from medical professionals should ALWAYS be taken priority over any content from this book. The author of this book, Andy Xiong, is not responsible for any physical injuries, physical health, or mental issues, including death, that may be caused by the contents of this book.

CONTENTS

Chapter 1

WHAT THIS
BOOK IS ABOUT

First, this book is 100% written by me, Andy X. I didn't hire any ghostwriters because I want every single word of this book to be coming directly from me. I want this book to be as authentic as possible, and I don't want anyone else to be my voice, so you can be the direct receiver on your end.

This book could drastically change your life for the better, and I can't wait to share everything with you.

My Philosophy

For most people, the physique of celebrities that you usually see in movies and on social media is their dream physique. Look good with minimal compromise.

For men, it's a muscular toned body that's not too big like those "scary" bodybuilders, not too shredded that every vein pops out of their skin, and yet have muscular definition and a visible 6-pack. It's that kind of body you'd see in movies and on models. It's what you imagine would look amazing when topless at the beach. Etc. Etc.

For women, it's usually that celebrity-like lean toned look, with hourglass curves while keeping the legs slim for a taller visual effect. They're not too lean to the point where that muscle definition begins to look too "masculine", yet they have those "three defined lines" down the abdominal area. Similar to men, that's an absolutely sexy physique you'd see in movies and on models.

For most people, they can imagine that only if they had that kind of physique, life would be great. They can just imagine that they'd have more heads turning, more romantic success, more confidence, feeling that they're just above the world, above the "average person" who is physically unfit and lacks energy. For most people, to have that body is only a dream.

Well, that was me. When I was overweight (which I was for the most part of my life), I could only dream of having that celebrity-like beach body. That people would look at me and envy.

And if you were also like me, and also imagined things this way, then you may have tried to get that physique. You may have tried to hit the gym, eat healthier, do more cardio, find all kinds of home exercises to do, go outside and run more, etc, etc. But if you've picked up this book, then I assume that, ultimately, nothing truly worked out for you, and you need some help in getting that dream physique.

Getting that celebrity-like physique wasn't as easy as you thought it'd be. (Well, it wasn't for me at first.)

2

But perhaps, you've got a bit more willpower than the average person. You put your head down and you grind it. And maybe you got some results... more than the average person, but probably still not quite like the dream physique you're after. But because of how difficult this was, you lost sight of what having your dream physique was for in the first place...

You wanted the dream physique so that you can enjoy life MORE with it, so you should feel that life is BETTER with it.

Yet it ended up that you had to be miserable to get even somewhat closer to your ideal physique. It was so difficult getting close to that physique, let alone keeping it. You realize that it's not enjoyable at all.

So here, I beg the question. If what it'd take to get and keep that dream physique is to be miserable for the rest of your life, then what's the point anymore?

That's like telling you to work a miserable job that you hate, working 20 hours a day, 365 days a year, with not much rest and sleep, no time to enjoy other parts of life, trading all that time in for a huge annual salary of $500K. And the catch here is that you have to keep working like this for the rest of your life, or suddenly all your money could be taken away. Even with all that money, if you can't even enjoy it, then what's the point?

Yes, I've realized this too, because I went through this exact experience, and had this exact thought process. I forced myself through the miserable process by eating "clean foods", "healthier" foods, doing lots of cardio - both HIIT cardio and running (which I absolutely hated), stuck to strict meal-prepped foods, ate "on time", etc. And with lots of willpower, I did in fact lose a lot of weight this way.

But I wasn't enjoying any part of it. And I realized that if that's what it takes to get and keep that dream physique, then there's no point anymore. Years ago when I realized this, I refused to believe that this was the end of the road. I knew there had to be a way to get that physique more effortlessly, and enjoy it too.

Today, I have the answer. And the answer to that problem is my philosophy.

The dream physique should be attainable while living a life in which we can effortlessly stay satiated and happy with the food we eat (without starving and being miserable), have an enjoyable way to train, and live such a life in which other areas of life aren't compromised or affected.

And if you believe that's the way you want to live your life while having that celebrity-like physique, and you want to learn exactly how to do that, then you're reading the right book.

What This Book Isn't, and Who This Book Isn't For

1. **This book isn't for people who are looking for a magic pill.** While I talk about this approach being "effortless", it's not ABSOLUTELY effortless (nothing in this world is). And it definitely isn't completely effortless

in the beginning to adapt. There is no "one trick", "one thing", or "a few simple things" that will magically get you the results. There are things you'd need to learn, and you must be open-minded about learning new science and the corresponding solutions.

2. **This book doesn't offer a shortcut.** While I maximize effectiveness and efficiency, it's by no means a "fast" fix. It requires a massive amount of patience. You'd better be good with delayed gratification. (Let me here break the news to you. Fast fixes don't exist anyway. So actually, the earlier you realize that and get on board with the facts that I'm offering you, the faster you'll get to your dream body.)

3. **This book isn't for those who are just here to criticize, and not here to seek actual guidance to change their physique.** Here's the deal. I've not only changed my own physique but also countless others who sought out professional help with positive attitudes. So the truth is, if you have great new science-backed information that counters what I provided in the book, I'd be happy to take a look. But if you're here to criticize, especially not in a constructive manner, I couldn't care less. Why? Simply because it doesn't affect my life. I'm here with one intention only: to share my knowledge and deliver (even over-deliver) value to the lives of those who truly seek it. So what you wish to do with your life, that's up to you. I don't really need to hear any of it.

4. **This book isn't for people who are closed-minded.** If you can't accept new things that are different,

sometimes even contrary to the conventional wisdom that most people believe in, then unfortunately I don't have any more solutions for you (you just have to accept being in whatever state you're in right now).

The reason why you're not fit is that you've already been doing things the conventional way that you were told to do. And look where it has gotten you! I assume that if you're already fit and have the body that you want in an effortless way, you wouldn't be reading this book. And if you keep doing what you've been doing, then you'll always be what you are right now and nothing will change.

So if you want the answer and want this to work for you, you must understand that most conventional wisdom is actually wrong. When most people go by that "conventional wisdom", you'll notice that they don't in fact get real results. Take a look at our world! It's no wonder that most people you encounter on the street are neither fit nor healthy.

And in this book, all of the "new" things are backed up by science (not only biological science, but in this book I'll be talking a lot about psychological science as well, because we all know that the fitness journey requires adherence, and psychology is important), so do rest assure that I didn't just make them up. They're simply different from what you've been told conventionally.

But I won't be going too deep into the actual science of everything, because this is a book for PRACTICAL solutions, not a science textbook. Plus, I think a textbook would bore most of you anyway. However, my approach will be based on science (I didn't get my degree of Medical Sciences and Psychology for no good advantages). **You don't have to take my word for it. In fact, I encourage that you don't - you should try things in this book for yourself, and do your own research.**

So, if we're clear on all this, and you're ready for real changes, then buckle up. It's time to transform your body, and your life.

Chapter 2

WHO TF AM I?

So you could be thinking, who the hell are you to tell me what to do?

If you don't care about my life story, and you just want to know how to get your dream physique and effortlessly keep it forever, then you can skip this chapter and go onto chapter 3. Otherwise...

My name is Andy X, CFP-PTS, DTS-1, BMSc, Hons BSc.

Yada, yada... Who cares. Letters ain't gonna help *YOU*.

Let me tell you the truth though. The fact is that, in the fitness industry, degrees and certifications don't really matter - because fitness is really in its infancy in terms of the entire industry. It's not as standardized and systematic as, say, medicine. And to be honest, most fitness "professionals" in the industry who have all sorts of degrees and certifications don't actually have a firm grasp of the real science behind fitness. So unfortunately, most of them can't deliver *REAL* results. That's the ugly truth. You just can't determine a fitness professional's competency with their degrees.

So I'm not here to impress you with a bunch of letters after my name. In this book, I'm here to give you real facts and practical solutions.

I'm here to talk to you like a real human (with scientific knowledge and methodologies).

This is me today.

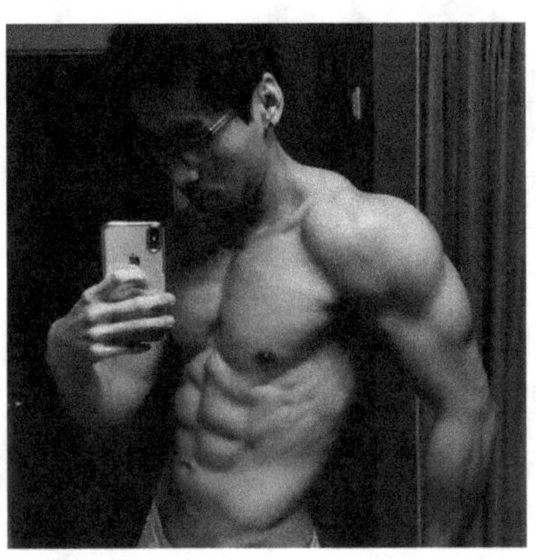

But I wasn't always like that.

In fact, I was fat for most of my life, ever since I came to Canada at the age of 9. High-calorie snacks and foods, along with a naturally huge appetite, and a Chinese mother whose knowledge in nutrition is anything but scientific, very quickly had me gain lots of weight. Within half a year, I became chubby. After another year or so, I became quite overweight.

So throughout high school, where your social life and self-esteem really began to matter, I was made fun of for being fat. I also wasn't very confident throughout my teenage years because of my appearance. I felt like I was the ugliest person that existed.

And that was reflected in being rejected by girls, which didn't help my confidence.

Then in my first year of university (in 2008), I began to work out here and there, tried to watch what I ate (I tried to eat "healthy", but as you read on in the book, you'll learn why that doesn't always work), and I got "some" results. But it wasn't anything close to what I have today, because I didn't have much lean mass, I became "skinny fat". And I got there through sheer forceful willpower, not through anything adherable.

So of course, I couldn't keep that up, and within a few months, I bounced back up in body fat. I went up to my all-time heaviest, at 214 lbs. (I'm 5'10", or 178 cm tall.)

I didn't take many photos because I wasn't confident to face reality. But here's one of the rare photos I took.

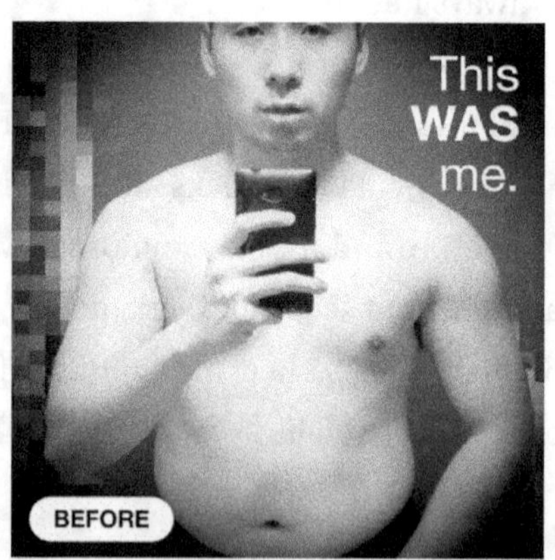

During that time, I had my first real romantic relationship. But because I was lacking a lot of confidence, I behaved in very insecure ways towards my girlfriend at the time. I couldn't even get myself to take off my shirt in front of her, because of how embarrassed I was for being fat! And I constantly feared that my girlfriend would leave me for someone else better looking. This ultimately drove her away, and left me in great pain.

Since that experience, I told myself I'd never want to feel like that again. I vowed to myself that I'll achieve a physique that will turn heads. That celebrity-like physique that you'd see in movies, that everyone admires - both men and women, young and old. A physique that's not just "kinda good", but close-to-perfection, with perfect ratio, clear 6-pack ab definition. A physique that's both powerful and sexy.

And so in 2010, my journey began.

In terms of both training and nutrition, I searched high and low, and tried everything. Literally everything I heard and saw. And back then, YouTube was still relatively new, and wasn't as filled with information as today. So in terms of social media, I was limited to channels like "SixPackShortcuts" (perhaps some of you may remember this), and scientific journals.

Speaking of scientific journals, I studied Medical Sciences (and later on, also Psychology) in university, so my background did help me in deciphering what information made real sense, and what didn't. I searched a lot of science journals in the area of nutrition and exercise sciences. But even then, the knowledge at the time was much more limited than today.

You may have heard of those outdated traditional BS info like, lift light in the 15-25 rep range to burn fat, or eat 6-8 meals a day to keep up your metabolism. (No. Those aren't true.)

With limited information available, I had to roll up my sleeves and do a lot of trial-and-error myself. I tried everything. Low fat diet. Low carb diet. No-carb diet. Detox. Pure-protein. Keto diet. Intermittent fasting. Paleo diet. Focusing on improving insulin sensitivity. Low this. High that. Anything you've seen and can think of, I'm 99% sure I've tried.

And just like that, I had no real results for 3 straight years.

But I never gave up. I knew there had to be a way. At least I learned what doesn't work.

Some time that year, during one of my full-body medical checkups, my doctor warned me that I had an over-active thyroid issue, meaning I had a lower metabolism than normal. She told me that I should try to lose weight in 6 months. After the 6-month period, I was scheduled for a follow-up checkup to see whether or not my thyroid improved. If not, I could be put under medication, or even surgery, depending on the root of the issue.

Well, little did she know, I had always been trying to lose fat. But now it wasn't just about how I felt about being fat, it was also affecting my health.

During that time, I had been already trying out intermittent fasting and counting calories. Fortunately, it worked, and I lost a lot of fat in a somewhat adherable way. Six months later when I went for my checkup, my doctor told me everything went back to normal.

That was a scare. But luckily I happened to have stumbled upon something that worked. So I built on that and continued to refine my methods. By then, I did build some muscle, and I did lose a lot of fat, but it wasn't absolutely adherable and the most efficient yet. It had a lot of flaws.

As I mentioned in chapter 1, I believed that there had to be an enjoyable way to do this. I refused to believe that having a mind-blowing physique means a miserable life.

Fast forward another year, I finally achieved a "good" physique for the very first time, in a way that was enjoyable and somewhat effortless for me. And throughout the years after that, as this began to be my career, I honed and perfected this method into a system.

Today, I've helped countless other individuals to also effortlessly get to their dream physique, while still being able to live out their preferred lifestyle and enjoy all kinds of delicious foods.

And truth be told, my physique has not only recovered my confidence, but it's now through the roof. I'm happy to report that I look at my body every morning partly to see how I can improve further, but a huge part is in the form of self-admiration. Not to tute my own horn, but it does put a smile on my face every morning, because I'm goddamn proud of myself. And I believe I've earned the right to admire what I've achieved.

By the way, as a byproduct, I can confirm that this kind of transformation does get you more (a lot more) attention from the opposite gender.

Today, I have the perfect way to get you there and stay there. And I can thank 3 things for it: determination, science, and common sense.

Determination... of course. I'm sure after reading my story, you should be able to tell that I was extremely determined, laser-beam focused.

The next factor for my success was science. Science is the study of becoming closer and closer to the "objective truth". What separated me from others was a solid foundation in understanding what real science is. Too many people in the fitness industry easily throw the word "science" around, but very little truly understand how it works.

And last but certainly not least, having common sense.

Most people when stepping onto the path of fitness:

1. forgot that they wanted to enjoy life better by having a better physique;

2. began to adopt the "bigger the better" approach, or;

3. not "open-minded" to try new things, and not realize that just because something was said by the majority at one time, doesn't always mean it's correct.

Whether or not you want to adopt that second point above, that's completely up to you. But I think that if you want to achieve your dream physique while not living a miserable life, it's important for you to adopt (the opposite of) the first and the third mentality.

Well, that's a little bit about me and my journey to physique success. I've walked the path once, so I got everything you need to get there, too.

Now it's your turn. Are you ready?

14

Chapter 3

THE MINDSET

I owe a lot of my fitness success to my mindset. And in this chapter, I'll break it down for you.

Before you start feeling a bit impatient now, thinking, "Okay Andy, just tell me how already", or think that this is just some hocus-pocus intangible BS, and decide that you should just skip this chapter, I highly advise that you don't.

It's because most people fail due to mindset issues, and the root of the issue isn't methodology. So if anything, this should be the most important chapter.

1   Know your "why".

Always begin with a purpose. It sounds like common sense, but believe it or not, in my professional experience, people don't actually do this.

Most people don't do fitness because they truly want to. They do it because other people and/or society told them that it's "good" for them, that it's the "right thing" to do for themselves, that they "should probably" do it, etc.

And none of those is because they themselves truly want to or believe that they need to.

And in one of the videos I mentioned on social media, I broke this "why" down to 2 types. Here I'll add 1 more, so a total of 3.

First, and in my opinion, the most powerful kind, is pain. Psychological science has shown that people do more to resolve pain than to pursue pleasure. And in order to feel pain, it must be A) great enough or important enough, and B) you have to have the sensitivity for it.

If the event or a consequence isn't painful enough, obviously you won't do much about it. But also, if you're not the sensitive type, to essentially "give a shit about yourself enough" type, then when a bad outcome occurs, you're going to have the "whatever, I don't care" attitude, which isn't helpful in this case.

So before all this, do give a shit about yourself. Know that if you don't, nobody in this world will care about you for you. You need to put your own matters into your own hands first.

And then, think about what matters to you. Do people make fun of you because of your physique? Does your romantic partner comment on it or care about it? Have you lost someone you loved because of it? Do you look in the mirror every morning or night and feel that you aren't living up to your potential? Find what is painful for you. Set the goal to eliminate it.

And if you have this type of "why", remember it.

The second kind of "why" is that you love the process. Unfortunately, if you've never done fitness before, you might not know if you love it or not. So this one could occur after you've tried for an extended period of time. But it won't be the reason to kickstart your fitness journey. But do pay attention to which part of the process you enjoy.

The third kind of "why" is ambition. If you're the type that holds a high standard for yourself, have the mentality of "I only live once, so why should I be inferior in certain areas of life", then you got the fire in you. You could have a great relationship, wealth, your dream job or the thing you love to do, why should that kind of life come with a mediocre physique?

Begin with your "why". It'll make the rest much easier.

2   Just do it.

The second step is to just do it.

I find that often the hardest part is not actually doing it. It's not even actually starting it. It's the decision to start, it's overcoming that stagnant comfortable state of inaction.

It's like pushing a heavy spherical boulder down a hill. When it's at the top of the hill, it rests comfortably. There are rocks and mud on the ground that keeps it stable. When you try to push it, it takes tremendous effort to get it moving at first. But once it starts moving, it begins to roll down the hill and will accelerate. And the amount of effort needed to keep it rolling becomes less and less.

Starting your fitness journey is the same. Everyone's got a little "comfortable person" inside them. That person will tell you "screw it, just stay home, it'll be much comfier that way". The more you entertain that little person inside you, the more persuasive that person becomes.

This is why you need step 1, to know your "why".

Then, you give yourself as little time to let that "person" speak up as possible. You just close your eyes, tell yourself "I don't give a damn", and just do it.

And the beginning will take some willpower. The good news is, psychological science will tell you that habits form with consistent action of about 1 month, and become solidified in 2-3 months. That means, as long as you just take action and do it for a short while, things will get easier.

So just think of it as "getting past that 1-month mark", instead of thinking of this as a really long process.

3   It's a road trip, not a grind.

As much as motivational speakers and "gurus" make it sound good by saying "it's all about discipline", "no pain no gain", we must remember (as mentioned in chapter 1) that our goal is to ENJOY LIFE MORE with a better physique.

I'd like to use going on a road trip as an analogy. If your goal is going from point A to point B is to enjoy the trip like a vacation, would you...

A. Drive from point A to point B as fast as possible, with no stopovers to enjoy the scenery, no rest points, drink lots of coffee so you can continuously grind it out? Or...

B. Treat it like an actual road trip, remembering to enjoy the scenery, plan rest points and interesting locations to check out, book a few hotels to rest up, take your time, and enjoy the ENTIRE way there?

I don't know about you, but option B sounds a lot more enjoyable to me.

Why would you treat the trip like some sort of mandatory mission, when there's really no deadline, and you can perfectly get to the same destination but in a more enjoyable way?

And the fact is, most people treat fitness journeys and the fat loss process as option A like there's some sort of deadline, and they're in a hurry to get there.

The end result of option A is that you'll hate it, and you'll unnecessarily grind out tremendous amounts of willpower.

Unfortunately, another factual consequence of choosing option A is that most people can't grind it to the end, so they can't even reach their destination. In the rare event that they do, by the time they finally arrive, they'd have no willpower left, and they just suddenly "let loose" and very quickly gain the weight back. Then here, I beg the question, why?

Why do it that way? Nobody assigned a deadline to you. You've got tons of time in your life to enjoy a great physique. Why did you have to get there in a few days, a few weeks, or even a few months? What's the rush?

When you treat your fitness journey and fat loss process as an enjoyable road trip, options open up and you'll find it much, MUCH easier to get there.

4   Don't underestimate the importance of your "willpower battery".

Earlier, I mentioned the word "willpower". An important concept that I'll be going into detail in the next chapter is, what I coin with the term, "willpower battery".

This is probably the most important psychological concept that most people, even most fitness professionals and "gurus", fail to realize.

This concept needs to be thoroughly introduced, so I've made an entire chapter dedicated to it.

Chapter 4

WILLPOWER BATTERY

W hen you think of a modern-day battery (like in a smartphone), you probably understand that:

1) It begins with a "fully-charged" amount of energy, and it decreases with usage and time,

2) It's limited in the amount of energy it can deliver,

3) Different ways of usage can result in different "drain rates" of the battery,

4) It can be recharged.

Your willpower works exactly like that.

What I'm about to talk about is backed up by psychological science. I'll save you from the tedious scientific explanation, and go right into how it works and what it means for you.

Imagine your willpower is just like your smartphone battery. For day-to-day willpower, you start the day with 100% battery. As the day goes on, along with the tasks you may need to do, your willpower battery is consumed. Near the end of the day, your willpower battery will probably be low and need recharging.

This is the **Daily Willpower Battery (DWB)**. The DWB can be recharged with sleep. This causes your DWB to begin at near 100% when you wake up in the morning, and low before you go to bed at night. Remember this pattern - it's extremely important for your success. I'll be talking about its practical usage later in the book.

DWB doesn't just apply to getting to your physique goals, but also shares with everything you do in your everyday life. For example, if you have a busy day due to work or school, and your primary priority in life are those tasks associated with work or school, chances are you're going to use your DWB for those tasks and worries. As you can see, in order to achieve your dream physique more effortlessly, it's important to understand how your DWB works and what you can do to minimize the use of DWB.

Then there's another battery concept.

On your smartphone, if you go into the settings menu, you can probably find a "battery health" stat somewhere in there. As the days go by, this "battery health" will decrease. The more you "take good care" of your battery and use your phone in ways that optimize battery health, the more your battery can last long-term.

When the battery health of your smartphone goes down, the "maximum" battery power it can hold on a day-to-day basis also decreases. After a year of owning your phone, you may notice that your phone battery drains down to 0% quicker than before, and it doesn't last as long as before. Your willpower is very similar.

This is what I call **Willpower Battery Health (WBH)**, which is the long-term condition of your willpower. The more you grind your DWB each day, the more your WBH deteriorates.

Here are a few things that would drain your DWB, and in the long term, hurt your WBH (and thus you SHOULDN'T do):

1 | Doing a type of training that you don't enjoy.

For example, if you're trying to lose fat, but you hate cardio, you do it anyway for the sake of fat loss. (See Chapter 18 for more explanation.)

2 | Restricting certain food items that you absolutely enjoy.

For example, if you absolutely love fried chicken, but believe that it's "bad for fat loss", so you force yourself away from it. When you see it on an ad, when you see a fried chicken restaurant on the street, or when you're with friends who are eating fried chicken, each time you restrict yourself from it, you're using too much DWB and grinding away WBH.

And even during times you're not actively restricting yourself, because you subconsciously have this "rule" that you cannot eat fried chicken, you're also grinding away WBH.

3 | Doing too much in your training. (I'll explain what this means later in the book.)

4 | Forcing yourself to eat foods you hate, just because you believe "it's good for you".

5 | Often draining your DWB down to none.

You may need to use your DWB for other important daily tasks, such as work or school. If you then try to use inefficient ways to lose fat and aim for your dream physique, you're going to ask your mind for more DWB than it has. If you do this often, it can hurt your WBH.

As you read on, I'll be mentioning willpower very often, because given that you're doing the "right" things, then preserving WBH is the key to success. I'll explain exactly what you should do in terms of training and eating in the later chapters. But for now, keep in mind the importance of WBH.

To summarize, DWB is your short-term willpower battery percentage. WBH is your long-term willpower battery health.

Chapter 5

THE PHYSIQUE

To get somewhere, you need to know exactly where your destination is. But if you picked up this book, most likely you're looking to change your physique into that lean, toned, sexy, celebrity-like physique (and do so in a lifestyle-friendly, "almost" effortlessly, and enjoyable way).

[IMPORTANT DISCLAIMER]

There is no one "best" physique. **I'm NOT advocating one type of body being "better" than others.** "*THE*" physique I'm talking about is based on what the majority find attractive on average and according to scientific findings. But you must remember that aesthetics is still subjective at the end of the day. Do what makes you happy! And often, you will find that most of the information you read in the book will still be applicable to whatever goal body you're after.

What the physique I'm talking about ISN'T:

- Bulky

- Bigger the better everywhere, disproportionate physique
- Skinny, but with very little lean muscle

Let's get into some examples.

For the gents, I think most people would like to have that lean, powerful yet not bulky look, and Chris Hemsworth, portrayed as Thor, represents that physique perfectly.

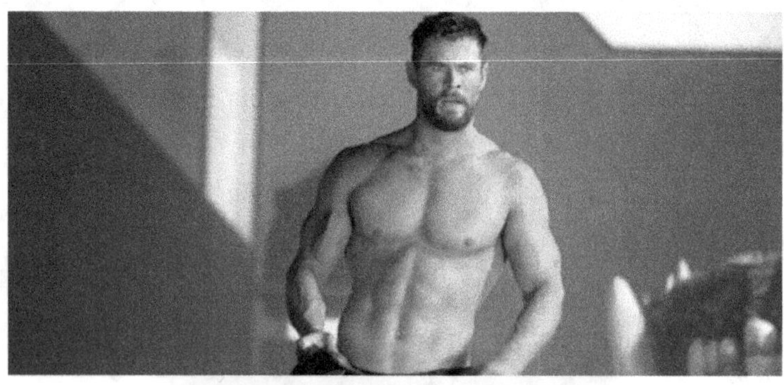

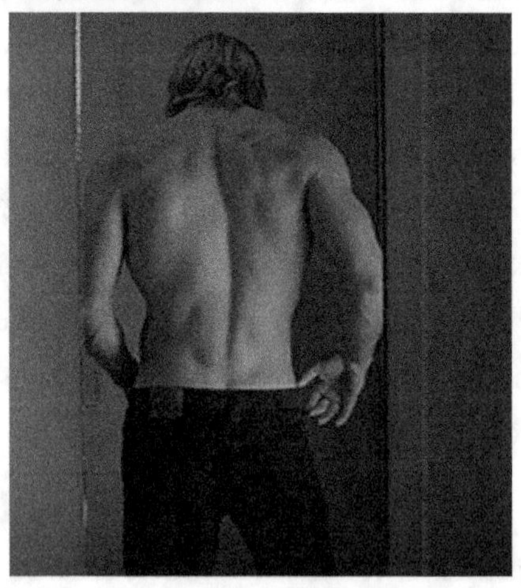

Let's break down his physique:

- Lean, has six-pack abs, but not vein-popping shredded
- Round, 3-D shoulders
- Wide shoulders, smaller waist - perfect shoulder-to-waist ratio
- Even-balanced, defined chest
- V-tapered wide, defined back

And for my Asian brothers, here's another example: Eddie Peng. Very similar type in terms of characteristics and bodily ratio, just less lean mass.

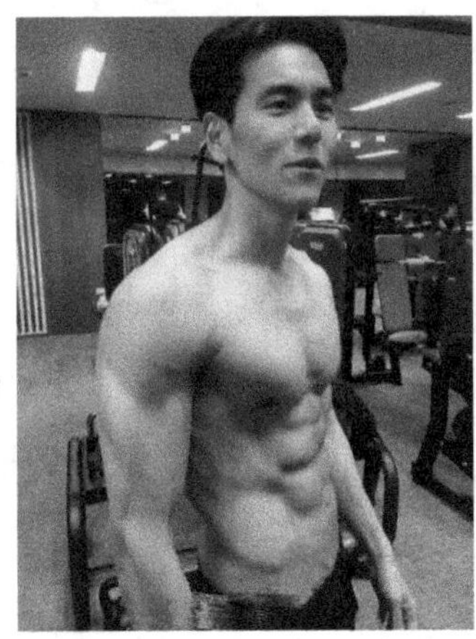

For the ladies, most are interested in weight loss. Although you don't want to look bulky, you can't just lose weight without any lean mass. A "skeleton wrapped in skin" look just isn't sexy. Kendall Jenner represents this perfectly.

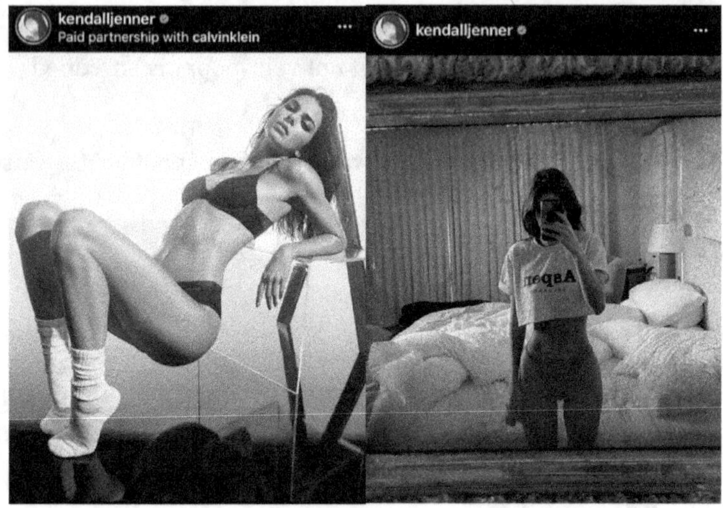

Let's break down her physique:

- Hourglass body, perfect waist-to-hip ratio - wide hips, thin waist
- Lean, has 3 lines down her abdominal, but not too lean that she has a full-blown six-pack
- A perfect thigh-to-calf ratio - too high would result in short-looking legs, too low would lose that sexiness
- A slight v-tapered back to enhance the thin appearance of the waist
- Defined back, but not bulky
- Defined arms, but not bulky

For the Asian ladies, here's another example. This is @nana.un from Instagram.

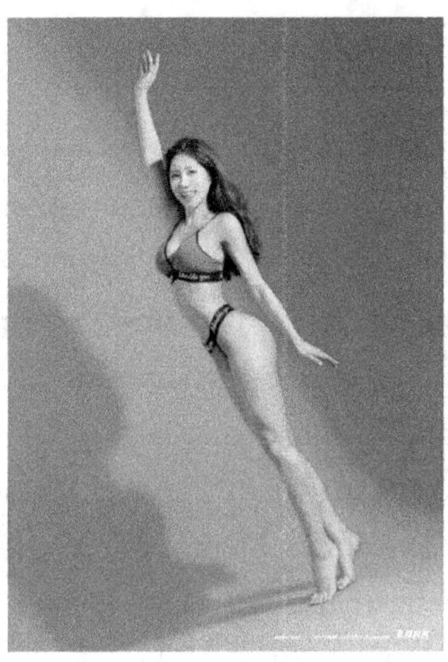

Although aesthetics is subjective, some of these human ratios are proven by science to be judged more attractive by the majority than others.

For example, a man with a shoulder-to-waist ratio close to 1.6 is judged to be more physically attractive by women, because they subconsciously believe that the man is physically strong.

For women, one with a waist-to-hip ratio of close to 0.7 is consistently judged to be more physically attractive by men (consistent in all generations), because they subconsciously believe that the woman is healthier and can bear healthier children.

Another point that we can observe is that all of these amazing physiques have one thing in common: they're lean and toned. Being toned means the body fat is low, so the muscular curves show through the skin, creating visible "definition".

So, having low body fat is key.

If we take a look at the ratio of lean mass (muscles) to fat mass, we can say that this type of physique all have something in common: high lean-mass-to-fat-mass ratio!

This concept in general is called **body composition**. And our goal is to "reorganize" our body composition, by 1) decreasing fat mass, and 2) increasing muscle mass.

But all in all, knowing what your goal physique is will be very important, because your training will need to be structured accordingly to sculpt that physique. You can't just do a bunch of cookie-cutter random training, thinking that just by doing some random movements or lifting weights will somehow get you to that dream physique of yours. There IS a science behind it.

Now, having your goal physique in mind, then there are things you need to add, and things you need to subtract from your body to get there. For example, you may need to lose the fat around your waist. Or you may need to add some size to your shoulders. But regardless of what your goal physique is, there are two LAWS that will apply to you:

1. **Subtracting mass (fat loss) is NOT done through training.** This is because you cannot "spot reduce" body fat - ie. you cannot pick which body part you want the body fat to come off from. For example, if you want to lose fat on your belly, you cannot do a bunch of ab crunches trying to lose fat there. Your body doesn't subtract mass by the specific area you train, but throughout your entire body.

2. **Adding mass (muscle gain) is done through training.**
    Where you add muscle is directly specific to the area you
    demand your body to exert force with.

You probably have heard that to lose weight, you exercise more, and eat less calories. Well, that's only part of the success formula, as you can see above. You don't just randomly exercise, and you cannot lose mass by primarily training (unless you're currently a professional athlete).

And knowing that it's calories-in-calories-out isn't enough. Everybody knows that eating fewer calories will cause you to lose fat, but if you take a look outside, most people still aren't fit.

Why?

Because there's still a learning curve to the process, there are still smarter ways to accomplish it.

Some people may know that calories matter, but not everyone knows how to apply it in an effortless, "just fits perfectly with their lifestyle" kind of approach. After all, "eat less move more" is definitely easier said than done.

So how do we do it? Without further ado, let's get started.

Chapter 6

FIRST RULE OF THE GAME: CALORIES

Science has repeatedly proven that the storage of fat is due to one reason: an **energy surplus** in your body. **And this is clear to the point that it's almost indisputable.**

Your body uses the food you eat as the energy it needs to function. When your body has excess energy from food that it doesn't immediately need, it stores away this energy as fat for later use. This mechanism developed in our bodies during the dawn of our species hundreds of thousands of years ago in order to help us survive - just in case we run out of food later on.

But in today's world, we pretty much never run out of food. And it's much easier for us to obtain. Because of this modern-day difference, our ancient survival mechanism is actually causing us trouble. When we eat too much food, we repeatedly store that extra energy as body fat, and accumulate that fat while never having the chance to deplete our fat stores.

Without the proper method to trick our body into using more fat and eating less energy, it's just difficult for us to achieve a net loss of energy with such abundance of food in our world. Our body physiologically screams "eat, eat, eat" in response to this overabundance of food, because we evolved in an era when food was scarce. That's why we have hunger signals and cravings. It's just hard to fight against our nature.

But having said all that, we know that the key to losing fat and maintaining a low body fat physique is to go on an energy deficit, long enough to deplete our body fat stores, yet also trick our body into feeling satisfied so that it doesn't keep screaming for food.

"So Andy, how can I eat as much as I want without getting fat?"

If you have a limited amount of financial income, can you spend "as much as you want" without going broke? The answer is, unfortunately, no, because money doesn't "grow on trees". So the unfortunate truth is the same for food. (However, there are smart ways to eat comfortably without getting fat, which I'll get into later on.)

Energy doesn't appear out of or disappear into thin air. This is the (First) Law of Thermodynamics.

"Energy cannot be created or destroyed. It can only be transformed from one form to another."

In food, we measure energy with the unit, kilocalories (kcal). In layperson's term, we simply call it calories (cal).

- If calories you eat > calories you burn (your maintenance calories)
  - You're in a calorie **surplus**
  - **RESULT: Weight/Fat gain**
- If calories you eat < calories you burn (your maintenance calories)
  - You're in a calorie **deficit**
  - **RESULT: Weight/Fat loss**

To calculate how many calories you should consume each day precisely, there are complicated formulas or other scientific processes to figure out. But luckily, for the purpose of body transformations for us regular folks, there's an easy way to estimate.

First, refer to the following visuals to determine your current body fat level. Then use these charts below to determine how many net calories you should aim for per day.

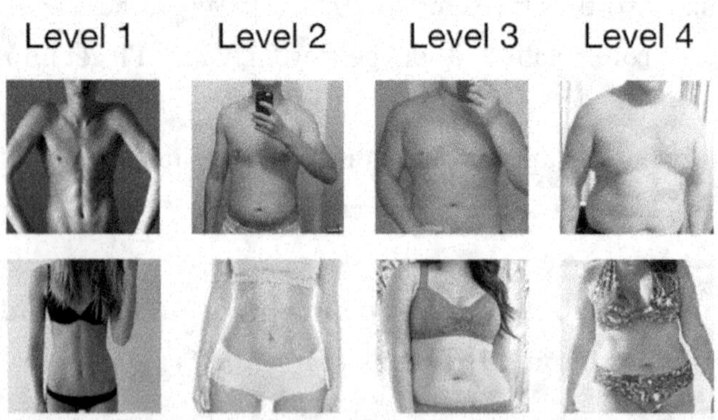

NOTE: *The unit for weight I use here is pound (lb). If you use other units, please do your own conversions accordingly.*

For Men

Beach body ab Definition?	Look fat?	Look muscular?	What you are	Net daily calories
No	Yes. Level 4	(Doesn't matter)	Overweight or obese	Bodyweight in lb x 9
No	Yes. Level 3	(Doesn't matter)	Chubby fat	Bodyweight in lb x 10
No	No. Level 2	No	Skinny fat	Bodyweight in lb x 12
No	No. Level 2	Yes, kind of	Average fit	Bodyweight in lb x 12
No	No, but a bit "puffy".	Yes	Experienced trainee, but not lean enough	Bodyweight in lb x 11
Yes	No. Level 1	No	Skinny	Bodyweight in lb x 14
Yes	No. Level 1	Yes, kind of	Lean and fit	Bodyweight in lb x 13, you're on the right track.
Yes	No. Level 1	Yes	Lean and muscular	Bodyweight in lb x 14. You're already good. What the hell are you doing reading this book for beginners? Just joking, you're still welcome!

For Women

Beach body ab "lines"?	Look fat?	Muscular shape and tone?	What you are	Net daily calories
No	Yes. Level 4	(Doesn't matter)	Overweight or obese (level 4)	Bodyweight in lb x 9
No	Yes. Level 3	(Doesn't matter)	Chubby fat	Bodyweight in lb x 10
No	No. Level 2	No	Skinny fat	Bodyweight in lb x 12
No	No. Level 2	Yes, kind of	Average fit	Bodyweight in lb x 12
No	No, but a bit "puffy".	Yes	Experienced trainee, but not lean enough	Bodyweight in lb x 11
Yes	No. Level 1	No	Skinny	Bodyweight in lb x 14
Yes	No. Level 1	Yes, kind of	Lean and fit	Bodyweight in lb x 13, you're on the right track.
Yes	No. Level 1	Yes	Lean and muscular	Bodyweight in lb x 14. You're already good. What the hell are you doing reading this book for beginners? Just joking, you're still welcome!

NOTE: *To calculate your maintenance calories, take your bodyweight in lbs, multiply by 14.*

36

For re-feed days (which I'll explain what these are later), take your **CURRENT** body weight in lbs, multiply by 14. Notice that it says "current", meaning this number will change as you lose weight.

Later on, I'll be using an example to make all of this clearer. But for now, keep in mind this chart. We'll come back to it.

FAQ: "I've been eating 'healthy', but I still can't lose weight. Why?"

This is a common question I get that just frustrates me.

The fact is, **your body doesn't care about how healthy you eat, when it comes to fat gain or loss!**

It stores fat when there's an energy surplus (from too much food), and withdraws energy from your body fat when there's an energy deficit.

THAT'S IT.

There is no second rule besides this.

Some "healthy" foods may have lower calories, so you could accidentally be in a calorie deficit by eating healthy foods. But there are tons of other "healthy" foods that are jam-packed with calories, such as avocados, nuts, and seeds. Eating healthy does NOT automatically mean you'll lose fat.

But first of all, what the hell is "healthy" food anyway? When "healthy food" is mentioned, many people immediately assume fruits and vegetables.

So meats are unhealthy? Now I'm not going to dive into religious beliefs. But for the rest of us who do eat meats, meats have nutrients that are essential for our health, such as a full profile of amino acids (protein), a high source of vitamins and minerals (that would otherwise be scarcer if you attempted to derive from other sources).

Then there are those "superfoods", like somehow eating those superfoods will make you instantly healthy. But the truth is, at the end of the day, sufficient nutrients in moderation is key.

As I'm writing this book, the current most popular "health food" is avocados. They are high in fats, which means that they are high in calorie density. I'm not saying that avocados are "unhealthy". But if you thought that just by eating healthy you can lose weight, and many people eat lots of avocados trying to lose weight, then you'll run into a problem - a difficulty in staying in a caloric deficit state.

At the end of the day, in terms of health (if you're currently healthy), 1) worry about being in a healthy body fat range first, 2) aim for a balance of all nutrients, and 3) don't think some foods are definitely "healthier", it's about moderation and sufficiency. But in terms of fat loss...

None of that even matters. It's simply energy balance.

I don't know exactly where the idea that "eating healthy automatically equates to fat loss" came from. Perhaps people associate eating healthy with being healthy, and being healthy with being fit. So they went ahead and linked that initial idea with the final ideas (eating healthy = being fit). Whatever the reason is, just stop. If you finish my book, and somehow you still hold all these false misconceptions, I'm seriously going to slap you silly.

Let's move onto the next topic. At the end of the next chapter, I'll be putting it all together.

Chapter 7

SECOND RULE OF THE GAME: MACROS AND PROTEIN

Your net calorie balance determines your overall weight change, but if you want that lean toned physique, it means you want to minimize lean mass loss and maximize fat loss, a higher lean-mass-to-body-fat ratio (also known as "**body composition**", as mentioned in Chapter 5).

That means you don't just lose bodyweight, you want your body to understand that it is the body FAT you want to lose.

Without telling your body that, you're not really "recomposing" that ratio. You're simply becoming a "smaller" version while your body composition remains similar.

So simply being in a calorie deficit isn't enough.

This is where macronutrients ("macros"), specifically protein, come in.

What are macros? In nutrition, we can classify our food into 3 "big" types of nutrients:

- Protein
- Fat
- Carbohydrate (Carb for short)

Now let's introduce the importance of each macro.

Let's start with carbs. These include primarily grains, fruits, and sugar. Carbs are important for 1) feeling good, 2) immediate energy (especially for physical activities), and 3) fills up your muscles to look fuller (if you eat just enough carbs and not too much).

Next is fats. These include all fats and oils, such as animal fat, fish oil, avocado, nuts, coconut, etc. Fats are important for 1) making food taste good (psychological factor), and 2) hormonal functioning. There are many other bodily functions that need fat intake, but hormones would be the main one.

Lastly, and arguably the **most important** for looking lean and toned, it's the protein. These include primarily meats, seafood, dairy products, eggs, beans, tofu, etc.

Protein is especially important, because:

1. Protein is the basic building block of muscles;
2. Protein signals your body that you need the lean mass, despite being in a calorie deficit, forcing your body to turn to other sources for energy;

3. Your body doesn't like to convert protein into body fat, even in a slight calorie surplus sometimes. Therefore, it's slightly more forgiving. (By the way, it's still not a ticket to a protein buffet without fat gain!)

So very quickly, you can see the importance of protein. It's the key to becoming and staying lean. **So definitely, we MUST eat enough protein.**

How much is enough? You'd generally want to eat protein (in g) at 0.8 - 0.9x your **GOAL body weight** in lb. Let's say, **0.85x** as average.

So in terms of the energy you consume, these 3 types of nutrients consist of pretty much all your intake.

1g of protein = 4 calories

1g of carb = 4 calories

1g of fat = 9 calories

That means:

Total calorie consumption = protein consumed + carb consumed + fat consumed + other calories (such as alcohol - usually not much calories is consumed in this category)

Assuming that there are no other calories than those coming from the 3 major macronutrients, then let me give you an example...

Let's say you're trying to lose weight. You're a 175 cm male, and you weigh 180 lb (chubby overweight). You'd be working with 1800 calories, and about 135g of protein.

On average, you'd find protein sources to be around 1:10 protein-to-calorie ratio (g/cal). A lot of foods actually have a lower ratio than that, because no food actually has 100% protein. It's usually a mixture of proteins, carbs, and fats.

So let's say you allocate foods for protein in terms of calories, that's 1350 calories in protein sources (if 1:10 ratio).

Going from that number, you'd have 1800-1350 = 450 calories remaining for other foods. So the fact is, it's not that many calories left! And if you wasted too many calories on foods that aren't considered "protein sources", you'd be in trouble trying to hit your protein target while still staying within your calorie budget.

So as you can see, given a limited amount of calories to work with, and **you MUST hit your protein target**, you don't want to waste your calories while not being able to get enough protein. That's like if you have a limited amount of monthly income, but you didn't plan your finances well, and you didn't allocate a budget to pay for your rent and bills. (You're going to run into trouble, because you won't have enough money!)

And it's the same with calories and protein. Therefore, it's important to make sure you hit your protein target by choosing a lot of your foods with a high **protein-to-calorie (P2C) ratio**. This is to make sure that you're getting the **best bang (protein) for your buck (calories)**.

A general rule of thumb is that if a "protein food" has a P2C ratio of 1:10 (for example, 10g of protein for 100 calories) or more, then it's considered pretty good. Usually, lean protein has more than a 2:10 ratio (20g of protein for every 100 calories).

In terms of how to structure your diet while hitting these nutritional targets to comfortably reach your dream physique, I'll be going into more detail later on. So keep reading.

FAQ: *"Isn't too much protein bad for you?"*

Science has shown that, for healthy individuals, protein does no harm to your body. In fact, a lack of protein is the key to muscle breakdown, which causes a cascade of issues, such as loss of muscle mass (which could lead to poor support for bones and joints), interference in bodily repair and recovery, etc.

However, science has also shown that protein is harmful for individuals who already have problems related to protein, such as kidney issues. This is because their kidneys are not functioning properly to begin with. For healthy individuals, this doesn't happen.

Please note that this book is for individuals who are healthy. Remember, if your healthcare professionals have advised you to follow instructions that differ from the information I'm presenting in this book, your healthcare professionals' recommendations MUST TAKE PRIORITY over mine.

FAQ: "Do I have to count calories and protein? Do I have to track my food?"

Obviously through your current natural ways of eating, you probably aren't happy with your resulting physique. I assume this is why you're reading this book in the first place.

So that means we need to do something different. And that's to troubleshoot and have certainty in our solution. I assume this is why you're seeking help. You want a solution that will certainly work and work relatively easily.

To increase the chance of success (to ensure certainty), measurement is absolutely necessary.

Imagine that you're running a business and wish to succeed. Do you think you can just arbitrarily "estimate" your finances and planning? Can you say "I'm too lazy to do the numbers for my business" and expect to succeed? Can you say "I just want to 'intuitively' run my business by simply going with how I feel" and expect to succeed?

Definitely not, and it'd sound silly to say that.

So you know you can't arbitrarily achieve great success in business without proper financial management. Then why would you think you can arbitrarily and easily achieve success in your physique transformation without calorie management?

What gets measured gets accomplished.

The good news is that calorie management isn't as hard as it seems. It isn't rocket science. The reality is that if you think it's a hassle, it's because of your own mental illusion. It's actually not much of a hassle once you get the hang of it. Calorie management is something you've never done, so there's a mental block that's causing you to feel like it's a hassle. So it's not the actual procedure that's causing the hassle, but probably because you just haven't even done it yet! It is simply this mental block, and that's the hardest part!

So what do you do? Refer to Chapter 2, the second point - "Just do it". Just like how I described it in that section, you will need to spend a little more willpower at first to create momentum. Then once the habit is formed in 2-3 months, then it becomes easy, and you just ride the wave.

"What if I still don't want to count calories and protein? Is there any other way?"

Then again, this book isn't for you, as I previously mentioned in Chapters 1 and 3. In Chapter 3, I mentioned that you need to know your why, and you need to "want it bad enough". If you don't, then maybe physique transformation isn't your top priority - which is totally fine. You should spend your energy doing something else.

Hopefully by now, we're on the same page. Now you should have your calorie and macronutrient targets calculated. I strongly recommend using an **app** (such as *MyFitnessPal*) and a **food scale** to learn to track your food. Once you get the hang of it, you can slowly move away from the food scale and even the app.

NOTE: In terms of tracking, you don't need to be bang-on precise with the numbers. For calories, track within the

ballpark of 25 cal. For protein, track within the ballpark of 5g.

Knowing your nutritional targets is one thing. How to go about hitting those targets is another. Most people know that to lose fat, you must be in a calorie deficit, but the majority of the population is still not fit, for a good reason. Staying in a calorie deficit for a prolonged period of time is hard for most people, because most people don't know the right approach.

You can hit the same nutritional targets, but with various approaches, such as different meal timing, choices of food, meal size, etc. Here in this book, I'll show you exactly how to find your perfect approach, so you can achieve your physique "almost effortlessly".

To succeed, you must know what some of the pitfalls that could cause you to give up are. Let's talk about that next.

Chapter 8

HUNGER, YOUR GREATEST ENEMY

By now, you should understand that to lose fat successfully and get to your dream physique, you need to stay in a calorie deficit consistently over a prolonged period of time. This is where the main problem comes in.

NOTE: If you don't need to be in a calorie deficit, then this may not apply to you.

The majority of the people who try to stay in a calorie deficit for a prolonged period of time end up giving up because of one common enemy: **hunger**.

When you're in a calorie deficit, your body simply doesn't like being in that state. And if you do it the wrong way, your body is going to stress, and raise its hunger level even more.

And you don't need me to give you that science jargon to tell you that hunger is a b*tch. The hungrier you are, the more willpower you need to resist. When your willpower battery depletes, you'd be on the verge of quitting. This is why most people quit!

By the end of the day, if you're still really hungry after using up all your calorie budget for the day, one of two things can happen:

A. You use willpower to force yourself not to eat, or;

B. You give in and eat, exceeding the calorie target, and no longer be in a calorie deficit.

None of the above are enjoyable and contribute to your goal. So we want to minimize hunger and keep it at bay.

There are 2 types of bodily signals that make you want to eat.

1   Hunger (Short-Term)

This is your daily hunger signal. Most people believe that you're hungry when your stomach is "empty". This is actually false in the majority of the situations!

Your daily hunger signals are actually synced with your internal biological clock. Just like when you get sleepy, your hunger signals depend heavily on time. This is why sometimes when you were too busy for lunch and didn't eat at the time you were hungry, beyond that "hunger time", you stopped being hungry, even though you didn't eat lunch.

How to keep it in check?

- **Protein-rich meals** provide satiety. So make sure you get enough protein daily and have some protein at each meal.

- **Adjust your meal frequency and timing**. Find the number of meals you need to eat comfortably. <u>If you have a bigger appetite, eat less meals. If you have a smaller appetite, eat more meals.</u> Adjusting your meal timing is much like adjusting your sleep time due to jet lag. You just need to fight the hunger signals initially, then your body will be taught its new meal times. I'll be going into details in later chapters on when and how to do this.

- **Eat foods that are less calorie-dense, so you can eat foods that are larger in physical volume.** This usually means slightly less in fats, because fats are the most calorie-dense macronutrients (1g of fat = 9 cal). This results in a bigger physical volume of food, which can keep you fuller for longer.

2   Craving (Long-Term)

Cravings are not short-term hunger signals, but the bodily signals that tell you that you're lacking certain nutrients or energy over a prolonged period of time. This isn't something you should ignore.

There are 2 major types of craving you should watch out for.

A   When you crave carbs

Even after eating a meal, you may feel that you're not hungry anymore, but not "satisfied". And you keep thinking of carb foods such as bread, potatoes, pasta, noodles, rice, etc.

This is because of 2 reasons:

a) You've been on a calorie deficit for too long, without any diet breaks.

b) You've been eating too little carbs for too long.

Your body has a hormone called **leptin**. Leptin is responsible for making sure you eat enough food for energy. When your body feels that it's been deprived of nutrition or energy (especially carbs), it decreases leptin level. When leptin is decreased, the food you eat becomes less satisfying, causing you to want to eat more. And we all know that this is counterproductive when we want to lose fat.

SOLUTIONS

1. **Maximize your daily carb intake, given the calories you can budget.** Despite most people thinking carbs will make you fat, it won't. Given that you can still be in a calorie deficit, you should actually eat MORE carbs, not less.

2. **Have "diet breaks".** Once every 2-3 months (usually when you're feeling like you're losing gas, and carb cravings are creeping in), you should take a diet break of 2-4 weeks. (DO NOT push yourself too much to the point that your leptin level crashes. Go on a diet break early.) During this diet break, you're simply eating at your maintenance calories. I'll be

going into detail on how to have a re-feed day in a later chapter.

3. **Have "re-feed days".** When your body fat is becoming low (for men, less than 15%; for women, less than 24%), science has shown that your leptin level is more likely to drop with a calorie deficit or a restricted level of carb intake. When your body fat is at this point, you should begin incorporating re-feed days, at least once or twice per week. I'll be going into detail on how to have a re-feed day in a later chapter.

B   When you crave high-calorie foods

... like pizza and burgers.

This usually happens for 2 reasons:

a)   You've been in a calorie deficit for too long or the deficit is too drastic.

b)   You're lacking fats.

SOLUTIONS

1.   Go on a diet break, like mentioned above.

2.   Incorporate maintenance-calorie days for a day or two consecutive days, with more fats and fewer carbs.

Final tip with cravings is... What you crave is what the nutrition your body needs. <u>However, it doesn't let you imagine the healthiest form of that nutrient.</u>

When this happens, break down the food you think about, and try substituting it with the macronutrients that food consists of.

So for example, if you crave for some candy, instead of eating sweets, try eating some whole-grain carb sources and fruits.

Tip: *If you got a sweet-tooth, try using a 0-calorie sweetener instead of regular sugar, as sugar makes sweet cravings worse.*

Now you're equipped with the knowledge of what to do when any type of hunger hits! When your hunger is minimized, you can stay in a calorie deficit consistently more comfortably. This is the key to success when pursuing your dream physique.

Here are some other tips to reduce hunger:

1. Drink plenty of zero or low-calorie fluids. It's not only important to drink plenty of fluid for health reasons, but it can also prevent you from being hungry frequently.
2. Go with your DWB pattern, not against it. As mentioned in Chapter 4, your DWB is highest when you wake up, and lowest before bed. So save up calories early in the day, and use the majority of your calories later in the day.

Next, let's talk about how you should choose your food.

Chapter 9

CHOOSING YOUR FOODS: CONSIDERATION POINTS

If you think, in order to stay in a calorie deficit and get lean, you should simply eat "healthy" or "clean", and it doesn't matter if the food tastes good to you, then this is why you ain't at your goal. The actual working method that's right for you isn't as simple as calories.

It's true that if you hit your target nutrition consistently, then theoretically you will get to your dream physique. But theory is one thing, applying it is another.

You're actually LIVING your daily life. It's not just numbers. That means your psychology will matter in the equation. If you choose your foods in a way that drains willpower, you're likely going to quit.

So the goal here is to choose your food so that you:

1. Hit your nutritional targets, and;
2. Make things easier for you so you aren't grinding out your willpower.

Long story short, you're working with a **limited** amount of calories.

So calories are precious, much like money. Make sure the calories you spend are worth every bit. People gain fat with poor calorie management, just like how some people accumulate debt because of poor money management. Fat = debt, and the price we pay for that is our health and life.

So with a limited amount of calories to work with, you really must choose how you spend your calorie budget wisely, so that you can not only be fit, but also enjoy your foods. Shall we begin?

"Wait Andy, so you're saying that I can just eat any foods I want, as long as I stay within my calorie target?"

Well, not quite. Going easy on your willpower doesn't just mean eating only the foods you love. Along with the P2C ratio that I talked about earlier, there are 2 more consideration points when choosing your foods. Let's begin.

1   Satiation

Ask yourself: "Does this food keep me full for a long enough time?"

Let's say your daily target calorie is 1600. If you were to spend 1600 calories on ice cream only, versus spending it all on chicken, vegetables, and rice, which way would minimize hunger?

Obviously the latter choice.

Like I said in the previous chapter, hunger is your number one enemy, because it can grind away your willpower (when you try to resist it due to calorie budget issues).

If you're trying to lose fat, you're already in a calorie deficit - something that your body doesn't like to be in. So make sure by the end of the day, you feel relatively satiated.

Let's call this: **satiation-to-calorie (S2C) ratio**.

One question you want to ask yourself when balancing the S2C ratio is, "How big is my natural appetite compared to the average person?"

If your answer is "bigger", then you might need foods with greater S2C ratios. If your answer is "smaller", then you could probably get away with foods with lower S2C ratios.

If you have a bigger natural appetite than the average person, and you ate foods mostly with low S2C ratio, you can probably imagine that you won't have a good time because you'd be hungry more often.

2   Happiness

Ask yourself: "Is the happiness level that this food brings me worth the calories I'm spending?"

Just like money, if you have a limited income, would you waste most of your money on things you don't even like? Probably not.

Remember, calories are precious, just like money. Spend the calories only if it's worth it.

For example, if chocolate cake only "kinda" brings you happiness, but you don't really care if you didn't have it, then don't waste your precious calories on that chocolate cake.

But if fried chicken brings you an absolute joy, and not having it for a long time would grind away your willpower, then this happiness is worth your calories. Then budget your calories to have some fried chicken in moderation.

Tip: *Consider substitutions if the happiness factor isn't affected too much.*

For example, if you love fried chicken, yet if you eat air-fried chicken, your happiness level isn't affected, then opt for air-fried chicken - because you can achieve a similar level of happiness with fewer calories.

But if you absolutely love the flavours of deep-fried chicken, and air-fried chicken just won't do it for you, then continue to enjoy some deep-fried chicken in moderation, as long as it's within your calorie budget.

It's about learning what you can sacrifice, and what you can't. Get it?

The point is, if you only went for satiation and have no consideration for happiness, then it can also grind away your willpower, because you're resisting the foods you love over a long period of time. Again, the strategy here is to minimize willpower wear.

This is why most people quit. They go balls-to-the-wall with their diet, eating only boiled chicken breasts and salads. And they end up unable to keep it up.

You're trying to achieve your dream body so you can enjoy life more. So what's the point if getting that dream body means you'd have to suffer?

So I call this factor, the **happiness-to-calorie (H2C) ratio.** You want to maintain a good level of happiness while balancing calorie consumption.

Let me give you some examples. If you compare a can of regular coke, versus diet coke, with that one swap, you could save about 140 calories. And in terms of happiness, the "decrease" in happiness by drinking diet coke is very much worth the 140 calories saved, because to me, diet coke doesn't taste that bad compared to regular coke.

But for another example, let's compare 100g chicken breast versus 100g chicken thigh - both skinless and boneless. The 100g chicken breast gives 165 calories, while the 100g of chicken thigh has about 180 calories. Eating the chicken breast would save me just 15 calories, but chicken thigh tastes WAY better. (Personally, I hate chicken breast in general, especially if prepared in ways that make them dry.) So in this case, eating chicken breast to save 15 calories is NOT worth the decrease in H2C ratio.

Taken together then, when choosing your food daily, you want to consider: is this food worth spending my precious calories on? Then consider the S2C and H2C ratios, as well as the P2C ratio (we talked about this in the last chapter). If you believe the answer is yes, budget your calories and enjoy. If you believe the answer is no, then perhaps you should stick with foods that will give you better S2C and H2C ratios.

FAQ: "Can you suggest some foods that I should be eating? What kind of protein sources do you suggest?"

Here I must stress this point. The entire reason why this approach works is because I'm not telling you exactly what to eat. You need to consider the P2C, S2C, and H2C factors, and eventually figure out what foods work best for you. For example, fried chicken works for me because I love it, but not everyone likes fried chicken as much as I do.

That being said, below I'm going to list for you some examples of protein sources in 3 lean categories.

P2C greater than 2:10 (Leanest)

- Chicken breast
- Turkey breast
- Most white fish
- Shelled seafood
- Lean cuts of steak (such as sirloin)

- Lean cuts of pork (such as tenderloin, loin)
- Extra-lean ground chicken
- Whey protein
- Egg whites

P2C between 1:10 to 2:10 (Very lean)

- Chicken (dark meat)
- Extra-lean ground beef
- Fried chicken breast
- Chicken wings
- Most cuts of beef (such as ribeye, striploin, brisket)
- 0-1% fat Greek yogurt
- Cottage cheese
- Most protein bars

P2C between 1:20 to 1:10 (Somewhat lean)

- Lean ground pork
- Lean ground beef
- Most fried chicken
- Most cuts of pork
- Pork ribs
- Beef ribs
- Most tofu and soy products
- Most beans
- Whole eggs

Now, here comes the exciting part now. ARE YOU READY FOR SOME SECRETS?

I'm going to share with you some of my best "tricks" as to how to decrease the calories of the foods you choose, while still being able to enjoy your foods. You don't have to apply every single one of these tricks, everyone has personal preferences, but you can certainly try them.

1. **Swap out sugar for artificial sweeteners.** This can be used with anything, from baked goods, to coffee or tea, to cooking with recipes that would otherwise use regular sugar.
2. If you have a sweet tooth, look for **low-calorie dessert options** (for example, there are low-calorie ice cream brands. Explore around). Try baking with Splenda. Alternatively, you can also try some protein bars, some of them can taste really good, with excellent calories and P2C ratio (generally 1:10).
3. **Cook with cooking oil spray**, instead of using actual oils or fats. Combine that with the use of a non-stick pan.
4. **Swap out fattier meats with leaner cuts** (while still considering H2C ratio). For example, pork belly and bacon are way too high in fats and calories, so I personally tend to use chicken bacon or leaner pork cuts such as tenderloin. But in terms of chicken, I tend to use fat-trimmed skinless chicken thighs over chicken breast, because even though chicken breast is leaner, it's not leaner by much, and thighs taste way better (way more H2C) for me.
5. **Invest in an air fryer** if you love fried foods.
6. **Try Greek yogurt (0-1% fat)** over regular yogurts.

7. **Swap out regular milk with almond or cashew milk.** They can be used as a creamer in your coffee if you'd like (gives it a great nutty taste), or can be used in cooking or baking where regular milk is needed.

8. **Use 0-calorie or low-calorie condiments and sauces** over their regular versions. Be careful with sauces that are high in sugar or fats. (It's NOT because sugar or fat can directly make you gain fat, but because they tend to have high calories.) Some good examples are:
   o   Hot sauces that aren't oil-based
   o   Soy sauce
   o   Vinegar
   o   No-added-sugar ketchup
   o   Mustard
   o   Greek yogurt (can be made into your own tzatziki sauce, or tartar sauce, etc.)
   o   0-calorie syrups (I won't mention which brand, but a quick Google search will give you lots of examples.)
   o   No-added-sugar fruit spreads
   o   Powdered peanut butter
   o   Low-calorie mayonnaise
   o   Dill pickles (can be diced and combined with other sauces to make a great condiment)
   o   Banana peppers
   o   Kimchi (for those amazing Korean dishes, or can be eaten as is)
   o   Seaweed (lots of amazing Japanese dishes, or can also be eaten like a snack)

- ○ Salsa

9. **Swap out whole eggs with egg whites.** You can find cartons of just egg white. Most dishes that require eggs can simply be swapped out with just egg whites.

10. **Find low-fat versions of foods**, instead of their whole-fat versions. Many foods that are high in fats are usually high in calorie density. For example, opt for low-fat cheese instead of regular cheese, or chicken or turkey sausages instead of regular sausages.

11. Most of us love pizza. So here's a bonus secret tip for the pizza lovers. **Try making your own pizza with a pita** (usually 0 fat) as the base, instead of regular pizza dough. Use no-sugar-added pizza sauce, low-fat cheese, and low-fat and low-calorie toppings. That's going to make a delicious pizza without the high calories.

If you apply all or most of those above, I'm sure you can keep the calories low while still being able to enjoy lots of delicious foods.

FAQ: "Aren't artificial sweeteners supposed to be bad for you?"

First of all, current scientific studies have not proven that artificial sweeteners "cause" harm to us. Most studies are essentially just showing their normal "toxicity levels" or the level at which harm could occur, but this is true for anything.

Even water has a toxicity level, meaning that there is a point which even too much water can cause harm to our bodies. Similarly in a lab setting, if a scientist were to inject water into a lab mouse at a level greater than it can handle, it will die. But it doesn't make water "poisonous" or "harmful". Artificial sweeteners are nowhere near the "toxicity" like that of cocaine or cyanide.

So relax. The bottom line is, artificial sweeteners are safe as of now. (By the way, I also hate how non-scientific media sources and some self-proclaimed "gurus" spread misinformation by "cherry-picking" and misinterpreting science. It causes unnecessary confusion and fear, such as on the topic of artificial sweeteners.)

As well, the word "artificial" may sound bad right off the bat. But if that's what you think, then I need you to hold off that assumption. This false assumption is known as **"natural fallacy"**, which assumes that anything natural is good, and anything artificial and "human-made" is bad. This is a false and oversimplification of the truth. For more detail, please refer to Chapter 19.

Now to put it fairly, that isn't to say that science in the future won't ever contradict this. We just don't know and I certainly can't see into the future. However...

If there were 2 options... Option 1, you use artificial sweeteners that are 0-calorie, so that it helps you control the calories enjoyably. Option 2, have the regular sugar and eat like the "average Joe", end up with a calorie surplus, and become overweight. Well, even though artificial sweeteners are safe "so far" but uncertain in the future, we know FOR SURE that being overweight and obesity DEFINITELY cause numerous health issues. So if you ask me, I'm going with option 1, any day of my life.

See FAQ in Chapter 11 for a detailed explanation of "Calories vs. Health".

Now, of course you can just not use sweeteners altogether. If that doesn't hurt your enjoyment of food, by all means go for it. But for me (and most others), the taste of food matters a lot in terms of enjoyment. So without sacrificing enjoyment, I'm going with option 1.

Chapter 10

INTERMITTENT FASTING

We talked about how going against your natural DWB patterns could make sticking to a certain amount of calories more difficult.

Your DWB is highest when you wake up, and lowest before you go to bed.

This means: You do NOT want to spend the majority of your calories early in the day when your DWB is high, but then when your DWB is low at the end of the day, you have to ask your DWB for willpower to resist that hunger. This would make things very difficult for you.

By working WITH that pattern, it means you save the majority of your calories near the end of the day when your DWB is naturally low. This makes sticking to your nutritional targets much easier.

NOTE: If your natural appetite is small to begin with, or you aren't in a calorie deficit and you feel that at the calorie target you're eating comfortably, then you don't have to use what's said in this chapter.

Deciding whether or not you should use Intermittent Fasting should primarily be based on how big your natural appetite is.

For example, if you're working with 1800 calories... if your appetite is big, you want to have bigger, but fewer meals. If your appetite is smaller, you want to have smaller, but more meals.

1800 cal					
900 cal			900 cal		
600 cal		600 cal		600 cal	
300 cal	300 cal	300 cal	300 cal	300 cal	300 cal

Now, if you're working with 1-2 meals, chances are you want to use Intermittent Fasting, because with fewer meals, you're going to NOT be eating (AKA fasting) during a part of your day.

The Problem With Most Fasting Methods

The first ideas of Intermittent Fasting came to popularity around the years 2010-2012. The most popular methods to perform intermittent fasting were the 16-8 and 5-2.

The 16-8 method means that everyday you have a 16-hour fast, and an 8-hour eating window.

The 5-2 method means that each week, you're eating at maintenance calorie or a slight calorie surplus for 5 days of the week. Then for 2 days, you're fasting the entire day.

Both ways could only work if OVERALL you're in a calorie deficit. However, here are the main problems with these two ways.

Remember, the goal here isn't just to lose fat, but make sticking to a calorie deficit (and therefore fat loss) an effortless thing to do. It's not about achieving it, but how you achieve it. Keep that in mind.

For the 5-2 method, your body cannot establish a firm biological clock around it. Your body tends to model a 24-hour routine. However, every week for 2 days, you must break out of that pattern and enter an entire day of fasting. This doesn't put your body in a comfortable state, making adherence harder.

For the 16-8 method, you don't have that issue. However, the main problem is its rigidity, falsely making the impression that timing matters a lot in this method. People fasted 16 hours with all their willpower, just waiting for that 8-hour "eating window" to begin. And when their eating window is "closing", they panic and try to get that last meal in.

This messes with people's lifestyles as well. They'd have trouble attending social settings when these events take place outside of their "eating windows", which can be quite frequent for some people. This clearly wasn't flexible enough to make things easy and enjoyable for people.

For most people, this created a binging cycle where people tried to stuff more food during the eating window, because they think that it's the only opportunity to eat. The problem is that calorie deficit is the main principle behind why it would work, and by eating past their maintenance calories (into a calorie surplus) during the eating window, they actually gained weight.

The bottom line is, when you set too many unnecessary rules around something, it drains willpower. These methods are meant to make things easier, but clearly they've made it harder.

The truth is, there's nothing magical about intermittent fasting. There's nothing magical about having a shortened eating window directly on fat loss.

How Should You Do Intermittent Fasting?

So now you might be wondering, what's my method of intermittent fasting then?

The key is, focus simply on the fasting duration after waking up.

Your goal is that at the end of the day, you hit your calorie and macronutrient targets, and you feel comfortable before you go to bed.

- If you still feel hungry easily when you go to bed, try pushing your first meal later in the day, and eating your last meal slightly closer to bedtime. You can also try reducing the number of meals by 1 and see.
- If you feel too stuffed when you go to bed, you can try eating slightly earlier in the day, and eating your last meal slightly earlier. You can also try dividing up your meals, and increase the number of meals by 1 and see.

In general, you'd fast 4-8 hours after waking up.

Remember, if with intermittent fasting, you're having a hard time eating all your calories by the end of the day, it means you got more calories to work with than your natural appetite. In this case, you don't need to do intermittent fasting.

FAQ: "Doesn't eating at night (eating late) make you gain fat?"

To reiterate, it's the overall energy balance that determines body fat change. Meal timing itself doesn't result in body fat change.

"But Andy, isn't your metabolism slower at night? Isn't that why you should eat more during the day, and less at night?"

While the metabolic speed can vary throughout the day, there's still a TOTAL metabolism for the day. So whatever your TDEE is, that already accounts for the varying metabolic speed, since it's called the "total" daily energy expenditure.

For example, let's say your total metabolism is 2000. And let's say during the day, your metabolism is faster, accounting for 1500 calories. And at night, your metabolism is slower, therefore the energy expenditure is 500 calories.

Let's take a look at the following 2 example cases.

In Case 1, you eat 2000 calories during the day, but nothing at night. In Case 2, you eat nothing during the day, but all of the 2000 calories at night.

Case 1:
Day Energy Balance = 2000 - 1500 = 500 calorie surplus
Night Energy Balance = 0 - 500 = -500 calorie deficit

So, Net Energy Balance = 500 - 500 = 0

Case 2:
Day Energy Balance = 0 - 1500 = -1500 calorie deficit
Night Energy Balance = 2000 - 500 = 1500 calorie surplus

So, Net Energy Balance = -1500 + 1500 = 0

As we can see, it doesn't matter when we eat, our net energy balance at the end depends on the total amount of energy we consume.

FAQ: "I'm trying out intermittent fasting, but I already get really hungry within the first 2 hours after waking, what should I do?"

Your daily hunger signals are mainly due to timing from your biological clock. Just like jet lag, you feel sleepy or awake, often not because of how many hours you need sleep, but because your biological clock hasn't adapted to the new timing. So, be patient.

In the case of fasting, I'd recommend that you spend a bit of willpower to get used to it. You do this by beginning with 1-2 hours of fasting after waking. And about every half of a week, you **add an hour to your fasting** until you reach your goal fasting duration that you ultimately feel comfortable with, as described above.

A tip to help you feel good is to drink plenty of zero or low-calorie fluids, such as WATER (!!!), sparkling water, tea, coffee, etc. Drinking moderate levels of caffeine is also a great way to suppress hunger, making fasting even easier. Moderate levels of caffeine are great not only for fasting, but they also help you focus during your fast and stay productive, as well as other health benefits.

FAQ: "Isn't caffeine bad for you?"

Caffeine when overdosed isn't good for you. However, in moderation, caffeine actually brings many health benefits. Here are some:

- Alertness

- Protects against cardiovascular attacks

- Antioxidant, protects against overall ageing and mortality

- Increases metabolism by increasing non-exercise activity thermogenesis (NEAT), which is extra movement that your body becomes naturally willing to do.

- Increases oxidation of fat cells - this means it helps your body unlock fat to burn

- Increases strength output in anaerobic exercises

- Increases endurance in aerobic exercises

FAQ: "How much caffeine is safe? How much is too much?"

First, everyone's different. One person may feel jittery after a can of coke, whereas another may feel nothing after 4 espresso shots. So the first and foremost guideline is to listen to how your body reacts, as everyone has their own personal tolerance.

According to scientific research, for the average person, the most amount of benefit comes from approximately 150-200 mg of caffeine daily. That's about 2 cups of coffee.

A single toxic dosage of caffeine is around 1000-1200 mg (~12 cups of coffee). But in general, you don't want to consume more than 500 mg per day (no more than 6 cups of the average sized coffee). Near this point is where the negative effects begin to come in. So unless you're using caffeine as a pre-workout stimulant (I'll talk about this later), stay under 500 mg. Caffeine is good for you in moderate amounts, but you don't need too much.

FAQ: "I've heard that we can only absorb 30-40g of protein in one go. But if I do intermittent fasting and eat fewer meals, I'd be forced to eat more protein per meal. Doesn't that affect how my body absorbs protein?"

While it's true that, according to research, muscle protein synthesis (building muscle) is at its highest efficiency if we spread out protein intake throughout the day, and only give our body 30-40g of protein at a time, but...

This decrease in efficiency is way too little, especially for regular folks just starting out. (This difference may be more applicable to advanced lifters, but even then... the difference is still NOT night and day.)

The fact is, if you ate ENOUGH protein overall for each day, even if you ate all of it in one go, your body will pace itself, and slowly take care of all the protein on its own. Your body is smarter than you think.

What's way more important is that we find a meal frequency for us to eat comfortably and meals are satiating, while still getting enough protein and staying within our calorie target. This is because by being comfortable, that's when we can do this consistently and effortlessly. In the long run of trying to build your dream lean beach body, consistency is WAY more important than trying to perfect muscle building (when it doesn't make that big of a difference anyway).

You see, intermittent fasting is no fat-loss magic. It's simply a tool for you to eat in a calorie deficit comfortably and enjoyably, by working with your natural DWB patterns.

Next, I'm going to sum up everything we've talked about so far, and take you through this entire nutrition planning process step-by-step.

Chapter 11

PUTTING IT ALL TOGETHER

Now that you have all the tools you need, let's go step-by-step as to how to plan and execute your nutrition. I'll also provide an example individual to take you by the hand and walk you through this entire process.

Step 1: Assess your current body.

Determine your current physique in terms of body fat level and proper training experience.

For body fat level, use the visuals in **Chapter 6** as a guideline. We don't need to be exact as to how much body fat we have in this step. Simply take a look at the pictures, and estimate which body fat level you fall in.

Keep in mind, for men, the first place to pack on fat is the **abdominal**, and then the chest and face, and lastly the limbs. For women, the first place to store fat is the **limbs**, and then the face, and lastly the chest and abdominals.

For "proper training experience", it's the number of years you've done some sort of proper resistance training. For most of you who've picked up this book, I'm going to assume that you haven't done any.

As well, use the charts found in **Chapter 6** for reference.

Let's use "Mr. Lean" as an example, an individual who's never properly trained. He's 24 years old, 175 cm in height, and 185 lbs in weight.

[Mr. Lean]

He looked at the visuals and believed that he falls in the "level 4" body fat.

Step 2: Determine your calorie target.

Use the charts in **Chapter 6** to determine your daily calorie target. Then round to the nearest 50.

[Mr. Lean]

His body fat is a "level 4", so he uses bodyweight in lbs x 9. That's 185 x 9 = 1665. Rounding to the nearest 50, that's 1650 cal.

FAQ: "Can I go on a bigger calorie deficit to lose fat faster?"

No, it's not recommended to go on a bigger deficit. Rest assured that the above recommended deficit is the most efficient and effective way to lose fat already. Once again, fat loss is simply your body drawing energy from your stored body fat. However, it can only draw energy at a specific speed (there are many factors that determine speed, such as hormones, current body fat, muscle protein synthesis, etc, but I'll save you the science here).

So by doing a bigger calorie deficit, it doesn't speed up the fat loss, but rather, because you've maxed out your fat loss speed, the extra deficit will no longer be coming from fat, but from muscles - which is pointless. You want to lose fat to look lean, not lose "weight". Muscle mass is GOOD, it helps you look lean.

Think of this as a dishwashing assembly line where one person rinses the dishes and the other person dries them. Both people do their tasks at certain limited speeds. By giving them MORE dishes, it doesn't mean they'll get more dishes cleaned. There's a maximum speed that they can work at.

Step 3: Determine the amount of protein you need.

Take your **GOAL** bodyweight in pounds (lbs), multiply that by 0.85. Round that number to the nearest 5. That is the number of grams of protein you need to consume daily.

NOTE: Your estimated goal bodyweight may change as you get closer and closer to it.

[Mr. Lean]

He estimated that his goal body weight is 160 lbs. Multiplying by 0.85, he got 136, which rounds to 135g of protein.

Step 4: Consider if you need re-feed days.

First, what is a "re-feed day"? On a re-feed day, you're eating at your maintenance calories: **CURRENT bodyweight in lbs x 13**. In terms of protein, you're eating at 0.8 times your body weight in pounds (lbs). As well, prioritize eating more carbs.

Check to see if you need re-feed days:
- If you're in the high body fat category, you don't have to take any re-feed days.
- If you're in the moderate body fat category, you must take at least 1 mandatory re-feed day per week.
- If you're in the lean category, you must take at least 1-2 mandatory re-feed days per week.
    - You should take at least 2 re-feed days (sometimes more) per week if you feel uncomfortably hungry very easily. Don't push your body too hard in this aspect.
- If you're not eating in a calorie deficit in the first place, then there is no need for re-feed days for you.

FAQ: "How do I determine when to take a re-feed day?"

So you're in the body fat range to need re-feed days. Here's how you should feel if you need re-feed days. Ask yourself:

1. Have you been in a calorie deficit consistently for more than 3 months and...

2. Are you experiencing (or beginning to experience) hunger where it seems like no matter what you eat, you still don't feel satisfied? Or...

3. Are you experiencing seemingly no fat loss progress for at least 3 weeks (like a fat loss "plateau"), when previously you were losing fat just fine?

If you answer yes to any of the above 3 questions, you should take a 3-4 week re-feed "period". You experience a lack of satiation from food because your leptin hormone has dropped. This is dangerous in terms of fat loss consistency, because hunger is the number one enemy to successful fat loss. So we MUST keep leptin happy.

By taking this re-feed period, this should restore leptin back to normal.

If you're experiencing a "fat loss plateau", chances are your metabolism has dropped slightly over a prolonged period of calorie deficit. To restore this back to normal, do what I recommended above (take 3-4 weeks of re-feed).

4. Are you going to spend time with your friends or family, or some occasion where eating at a calorie deficit would be difficult without sacrificing enjoyment? Or...

5. Do you just want to eat at maintenance calories, to take a break?

If you answer yes to questions 4 and 5, then go ahead and take a re-feed day. There are no mandatory rules saying you must eat at a calorie deficit every single day. (See the next FAQ below for more explanation.)

FAQ: *"Will I get fat if I take too many re-feed days?"*

No, you won't get fat. On a scale, you may see weight fluctuations. But rest assured that it's not fat gain. In fact, it's just taking a break from being on a constant deficit. Refer to the mindset "road trip" in Chapter 3.

Tip: You can plan your re-feed days on days that you might eat a bit more, such as weekends as days you know you're going out with friends or family. This way, you'll have more calories to work with and have a more enjoyable time.

Sometimes, you can even take a few more days of re-feeds by going on maintenance calories. Remember that eating at maintenance calories will only solidify your current body, and will not make you gain fat. So just like a road trip, it's okay to take a "break" for a while if you need it. Nobody is racing you to get lean, so take your time!

FAQ: *"Is re-feed day like a cheat day?"*

Absolutely not.

When you think about "cheat day", you probably think that it's a day where you "let loose". But my question is, what's there to "let loose" if you're not that miserable eating with this method in the first place? A cheat day is an escape. With my method here, you won't feel like you have to escape. A re-feed day is part of a planned strategy. (I'll explain that very soon.)

As well, if you feel like you want to eat more carbs, or eat a bit more in general while you're on a calorie deficit, feel free to take more re-feed days until you feel better.

[Mr. Lean]

He's in the high body fat category, so he doesn't have to take any re-feed days. But if he does, then he would eat at maintenance calories (calculated by **taking CURRENT weight in lbs, multiply by 13**). In terms of protein, multiply 160 (his body weight in pounds) by 0.8, which is 128, rounded to 130g of protein.

Step 5: Choosing your foods.

Calories are precious, because you only have a limited amount of calories to work with. So it's important to choose foods that make your life easier and more enjoyable.

The ideal here is that, because the calories you are working with are limited, you need to spend your calories wisely - balance the P2C, H2C, and S2C ratios (we talked about these in the previous chapters). This step is a lifetime evaluation where you'll need to constantly observe and modify your evaluation.

Just like a financial investment - you want to think about the "return on investment (ROI)" - what is the P2C, H2C, and S2C **return on caloric investment (ROCI)** for the calories you spend?

Here are the questions you want to ask yourself:

1. What are some of your favourite foods that you absolutely cannot sacrifice? Consider their P2C and S2C ratios.

2. What are some of your favourite protein sources? Consider their P2C and H2C ratios.

3. What are some foods you love, but feel like you'll be fine if you didn't have them very often? (These are the foods you can swap out, or could try their lower-calorie alternatives.)

4. How is your natural appetite compared to the average person? More or less? (This question is important, as mentioned in Chapter 8.)

[Mr. Lean]

- His absolute favourite foods are fried chicken, chocolate ice cream, and bubble tea.
    - Fried chicken has a decent P2C ratio because chicken is high in protein, and it's also very satiating. H2C is extremely high.
    - Chocolate ice cream has almost no protein, so its P2C ratio is low. Its S2C ratio is also low because it's not satiating at all. But he loves chocolate ice cream way too much to give it up, so the H2C is extremely high.
    - Bubble tea also has a low P2C and S2C ratio. Initially, he thought it brought him extreme happiness. But over time, as he realizes that he doesn't have many calories to work with if he drank too much bubble tea, he began to feel that he could sacrifice bubble tea,

because it didn't bring him as much happiness as he previously thought. (Eventually, he gave up bubble tea.)

- His favourite protein source is chicken. Within his calorie budget, he can also enjoy some fried chicken in moderation.
- He loves milky beverages, such as bubble tea and coffee with cream.
  - But he realizes that it's not as mandatory as other foods such as fried chicken and ice cream.
  - He swaps out bubble tea for non-cream tea such as oolong and Japanese green tea. H2C is maintained high because the calories in these teas are 0, while he still enjoys these swaps.
  - He swaps out the cream with almond milk in his coffees. This drastically reduced the calories, while the happiness didn't decrease by much for him. So H2C is still maintained high.
- Within his calorie budget, he frequently enjoys fried chicken because its P2C and S2C ratios are still pretty decent. However, he only enjoys some chocolate ice cream once a week, because both P2C and S2C ratios are low. However, he understands that he isn't restricting his food choices, so he comes to terms with this moderation.
- His appetite size is greater than that of the average person. So he has to make sure more foods he eats are higher in

the S2C ratio, and enjoy foods low in S2C ratio less frequently (such as ice cream).

Step 6: Plan your meal frequency and timing.

This mainly depends on 2 factors:

1. Whether or not you're in a calorie deficit or not;
2. Your natural appetite.

1   Are you in a calorie deficit?

If the answer is yes, then in general, you want to reduce your meal frequency and push your first meal later after you wake up. In some cases, if you don't have that many calories to work with, you could reduce your daily meal frequency to 1 or 2. In general, you would want to spend more calories near the end of your day, and fewer calories at the beginning of your day.

If your answer is no, then it depends on the next factor.

2   How big is your natural appetite?

Do you find yourself having bigger or smaller than the average person's appetite?

If your answer is "smaller", then you want to increase your meal frequency, and begin your first meal earlier in the day.

If your answer is "bigger", then you want to reduce your meal frequency to allow bigger meals, and begin your first meal later in the day. Also, you want to spend fewer calories at the beginning of the day, and most of your calories at the end of the day.

(Refer to Chapter 10 for a more detailed explanation.)

Why? Because of the nature of the Daily Willpower Battery (DWB).

If your natural appetite is big, you're more likely to run into hunger issues. As mentioned in Chapter 4, your DWB is highest when you wake up, and lowest before bed.

So you shouldn't work AGAINST the pattern. You do NOT want to spend the majority of your calories early in the day when your DWB is high, but then when your DWB is low at the end of the day, you have to grind out the rest of your DWB resisting that hunger.

By working WITH that pattern, it means you save the majority of your calories near the end of the day when your DWB is naturally low. This makes sticking to your nutritional targets much easier.

As mentioned in Chapter 10, if you find yourself easily running into hunger issues, an incredible tool is the Intermittent Fasting strategy.

[Mr. Lean]

He is in a calorie deficit. And because his natural appetite is big, he needs bigger meals to feel satisfied. So he reduced his meal frequency to 2 times per day.

Also, he does intermittent fasting to further help him stay satisfied on a calorie deficit. He wakes up at 7 am for work, doesn't eat until 6 hours later, which is 1 pm. During his fast, he drinks plenty of water. At around 11 am, he usually enjoys a cup of black Americano coffee. Then at 1 pm, he usually enjoys a light lunch using about 400-600 calories.

At 7 pm, he usually enjoys a big dinner using about 800-1000 calories with his family.

Before bedtime (at around 10 pm), if he occasionally has unused daily calories remaining, he will enjoy a scoop of chocolate ice cream (~150 calories).

FAQ: "Is it mandatory for me to hit my calorie target if I want to get results?"

To get good results, it's RECOMMENDED to aim for the calorie deficits I mentioned earlier, because that's the **most** efficient speed you COULD go.

But it's not mandatory. The fact is, as long as you're in a calorie deficit, it doesn't matter how small it is, you will still lose fat. It's only a matter of speed. You can go slower if you want to.

Mr. Lean hits his nutritional target 95% of the time. The few times he doesn't, he doesn't worry too much about it. His maintenance calorie is 2200. His daily goal is 1550. However, if one day he ate a bit more and hit 1700 cal (for example), he doesn't need to beat himself up over it because 1700 is still under 2200, which means he is still losing fat.

As long as Mr. Lean doesn't consistently eat over 2200 cal, he won't be gaining any significant amount of fat, he won't be ruining his progress.

FAQ: "All you've mentioned are calories and protein. But what about health?"

Good question.

Many people demonize calorie-counting and think that "all they care about is calories, it doesn't mean good health". And this idea is simply not true.

According to the World Health Organization, the number one cause of death is heart disease. In Canada, heart disease is number two. **And the leading risk factor for heart disease is obesity.**

Along with the risk of heart disease, being overweight is a huge risk factor for countless other issues of both physical and mental health. Off the top of my head, I can already list a few: type-2 diabetes, thyroid-related illness, joint damage (such as the knee, hip, ankle, etc.), eating disorders, mental issues (depression, low self-esteem, etc.) related to body image, dementia, many types of cancer, etc. The list goes on.

And here's the cold-hard truth. Obesity is not a disease you catch. Obesity is the outcome of accumulated poor nutrition decisions. **Obesity is the result of accumulated calorie surplus over a long period of time.**

So calorie management is in fact THE MOST IMPORTANT thing you can do that's related to general health, in (literally) the reduction of your death probability.

The fact is...

YOU CANNOT SEPARATE WEIGHT CONTROL FROM HEALTH.

Calorie management is a giant part of good practise of health.

As well, let's talk about aging - the "ultimate" death.

The reason why we "age" is because of the "oxidation" that happens in our cells. I'll save you the science, but long story short, as the cells in our body work to convert your food into energy, it produces "oxygen free radical" as a byproduct.

When a cell has too many free radicals, it leads to death of that cell. For your body as a whole, the more your cells do this, the more we "age".

You've probably heard of foods containing antioxidants or antioxidant supplements, which are things that help slow down this oxygen free radical production. However, no matter how much antioxidants you have to "slow down aging", **the fact is that the more calories you consume, the more aging happens.**

Yes. Consuming more calories is literally killing you.

Think of your body like a car. The more mileage you put on your car, the more likely it is for your car to have issues and ultimately break down. Calories are like the mileages on our body.

So there you have it. I've just given you two huge reasons why calorie management is one of the most important things you need to do for better general health.

It is true that calories aren't the ONLY thing for good health. **Getting sufficient micronutrients (vitamins and minerals) is also important.** So make sure you're spending some of your calorie budget on some fruits and plenty of vegetables, as well as a wide variety of other foods to make sure you're getting a wide range of micronutrients.

Chapter 12

THE COMMON MYTHS OF METABOLISM

There's been a lot of confusion surrounding metabolism. Fitness and "health" industries and "gurus" spreading these familiar words:

- You can trick your body into boosting its metabolism.
- You can't lose weight because of "slow metabolism".
- Here are the top 10 "superfoods" that will "boost" your metabolism and help you lose fat.
- Start your day with a breakfast that'll "kickstart" your metabolism so you can start losing fat immediately.
- Eat every 2-3 hours to "keep your metabolism high" to lose fat.

If you've heard these before, then let me mute the noise and give you the REAL truth.

All of the above are false. Yes. All.

Read on, and you'll understand very soon. But first, we must define what metabolism is.

What is metabolism?

Metabolism is simply anything and everything your body does. This includes withdrawing energy from your fat stores, building muscles, regulating heartbeat, your conscious and subconscious brain activities, exercising, walking... making sperm!

Literally. Everything.

Now, as far as we regular folks are concerned, for our purpose of losing fat, getting in shape, building some muscles, toning our body, etc... we don't really care about the actual science...

For us, **metabolism is the total ENERGY your body needs to do everything it does.**

What's really included in this "metabolism"?

Metabolism, as professionals call it **Total Daily Energy Expenditure (TDEE)**, is made up of a lot of processes. As far as we're concerned, we need to deal with only the biggest chunks of your metabolism, as they affect our fitness and fat loss process the most.

Here's what metabolism includes:

Metabolism = Resting Metabolic Rate (RMR) + Thermic Effect of Food (TEF) + Thermic Effect of Activities (TEA) + Non-Exercise Activity Thermogenesis (NEAT)

RMR: The LEAST amount of energy you need to maintain your body while you externally do absolutely nothing. This is affected by 1) genetic factors, such as height and gender, 2) current weight ("what your body is made of, and how much").

TEF: The energy you need to digest and breakdown food.

TEA: The energy you need to do intentional physical activities.

NEAT: The energy you need to do everything other than intentional physical activities (such as walking, or as little as an unconscious movement like fidgeting).

Here's a rough breakdown in a pie chart what it looks like.

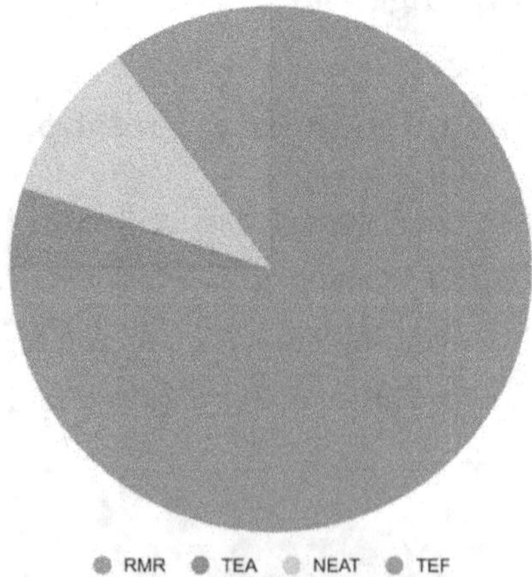

How does this apply to fat loss?

Immediately what you notice above is that the largest chunk of your metabolism is **RMR (~75% of your TDEE), NOT physical exercises (~5-10%)**. Remember this. This is extremely important to recognize.

Now, I stress this point once again. **The overarching law that governs above all other concepts is energy (calories).** NOT insulin, NOT genetics, NOT carbs, etc etc.

So in order to lose fat, the total amount of calories you consume must be LESS than the energy that your metabolism needs. To reiterate from Chapter 6, this is called a calorie deficit.

Now some of you may wonder...

"Hey, if that's true, instead of decreasing what I eat, can't I increase my metabolism?"

Even though mathematically and logically, that makes sense, let me share with you the truth on that. This brings us to the next topic.

Can you increase my metabolism?

First of all, it's important to understand that, as far as we're concerned:

1. **Your RMR (given a certain current body weight) is largely determined by your genetics.**
   So you can't change your innate metabolism, nor can

you "speed up" or "slow down" that metabolism to any significant extent.

2. **The calories you eat (on the "what you eat" side of the equation) will ALWAYS be greater than the Thermic Effect of Food (TEF) (the "what you burn" side of the equation).**

   That means, you can't boost your metabolism to the extent that you can rely on it to create a deficit. Your TEF will **never** catch up to the actual calorie content of the food you eat.

3. While you could "control" TEA and NEAT, on a practical level, there is a HUGE catch to this. **So it's NOT as simple as, "do more cardio/exercises to burn more calories".**

But we need to be clear on one thing. According to the 3 points above, we can see that **THERE ARE NO TRICKS TO BOOSTING YOUR METABOLISM.** Let's revisit a few ideas mentioned in the beginning.

IDEA 1: You can trick your body into boosting its metabolism.

True or false? **FALSE.**

FACT: You can only "increase your metabolism" by increasing the need for energy, literally by more physical movement, as we can see in point 3 above.

People treat our bodies like some sort of separate entity, as if we can somehow manipulate it. But the truth is... we ARE LITERALLY our body.

The fact is, in order for our body to burn more energy, we have to literally do more work (whether that's internally in your body or externally by actually moving around). There are no magic pills or shortcuts here. To burn more calories, WE need to do more work in proportion.

IDEA 2: You can't lose weight because your metabolism has crashed/slowed down.

True or false? **FALSE**.

FACT: As we can see in the calorie deficit idea, as long as we eat less than our metabolism, we can ALWAYS lose fat, regardless of such "slowdown".

As well, except at the extremely rare chance that you have some sort of metabolic disorder (which you need to seek medical professionals for help, not here), your metabolism isn't low. In fact, it's determined by genetics (as mentioned in point 1 above), and your natural **range** of metabolism is pretty much set in stone.

IDEA 3: Here are the top 10 "superfoods" that will "boost" your metabolism, and help you lose weight.

True or false? **FALSE**.

FACT: As mentioned in point 2 above, you can NEVER burn more calories by digesting the food than the calories you eat from the same food. Therefore, even though by eating more food, yes you're spending more energy digesting, but you're also accumulating more calories into your body.

So no. You cannot lose weight by eating MORE calories (even the so-called "superfoods").

IDEA 4: Start your day with a big breakfast that'll "kickstart" your metabolism, which will help you start burning fat as early as possible.

True or false? **FALSE.**

FACT: Same as the previous idea.

IDEA 5: Eat every 2-3 hours to "keep your metabolism high'.

True or false? **FALSE.**

FACT: Your metabolism, as far as we're concerned, is the AMOUNT, not the speed. The speed is more or less set in stone by genetics.

By eating more frequently, you're simply accumulating more calories in the "what you eat" side, and thus reduces the likelihood of you being in a calorie deficit.

Same as IDEA 3, you cannot lose weight from burning more calories by digesting. You cannot lose weight by eating MORE calories.

So coming back to the question, "Can I increase my metabolism?"

The answer is, **NO - not to the extent that you can rely on it for fat loss.**

"But Andy, what about exercising and cardio? Doesn't that burn more calories?"

Mathematically yes. But the difference isn't significant, nor practical.

If you go back to the pie chart of the TDEE breakdown earlier, remember that exercising on average doesn't contribute to any significant proportion in your overall TDEE.

And hormonally, it's also less practical. Previously, I've mentioned the hormones that we need to worry about. **Long story short, if you're doing cardio PURELY for the sake of fat loss, then it's not worth it.**

Your body isn't a static mathematical robot. It's a complex dynamic biological machine.

When you do moderate to intense cardio (especially one that you hate), in general:

1. **Your stress hormone, cortisol, goes up**. This causes your body to slow down a lot of its other bodily functions and causes it to hold onto your body fat more. Why? Because it's getting ready to repair your body from the aftermath of your cardio workout.

2. **Your satiation hormone, leptin, goes down.** ESPECIALLY during fat loss, you want your precious leptin to be kept high up! Lower leptin = more eating

needed to feel full. This would jeopardize the likelihood for you to stay in that calorie deficit.

3. **Your hunger hormone, ghrelin, goes up.** Self-explanatory. After excessive cardio, your body now needs energy back in, so your hunger hormone shoots up.

4. **Your willpower goes down.** This is VITAL in fat loss because the depletion of willpower is when you quit your fat loss pursuit.

(See Chapter 19 for more detailed explanation.)

Keep in mind that, **instead of focusing on what shortcuts** you can use to "boost" your metabolism, **focus on your actual diet and nutrition instead, and make sure you're in a CALORIE DEFICIT.**

What about the metabolic crash people talk about? Is it true?

As you stay in a proper calorie deficit (10-25% deficit) for a prolonged period of time, you may notice your weight drop. However, as you lose more and more weight, you may notice that your fat loss progress seems to "slow down", and "plateaus". So what's really happening there? Did your metabolism really crash?

The truth is, there was a drop in metabolism - but hardly a "crash". When we say "crash", we indicate something severe, like it has dropped SIGNIFICANTLY. But that's NOT the case here.

However, the MAJORITY of the reason why your metabolism dropped is simply because... **there's less of you!** That's the main reason.

When your weight drops, your body essentially has less "stuff". As we mentioned earlier, one factor that determines your RMR is body weight. **So if your weight changes, so does your RMR.**

So what really happened was that your RMR dropped, and **it partially cancelled out your deficit that you initially were trying to put in place.**

But is that it? Does your metabolism drop due to hormonal reasons (excluding the drop due to your body weight decrease)?

Yes, it does - BUT does it cause you to stop losing weight? The answer is: not to any significant extent, as **calorie deficit is STILL the overarching law of fat loss.**

Science has shown that when you diet down to a lower body fat (prolonged period of calorie deficit), many of your bodily functions begin to slow down. And this is all due to your body trying to survive. (It's a survival machine!)

Hormonally, your stress hormone, cortisol, will go up. And your satiation hormone, leptin, will go down. The end result is that you won't feel good, and you're always hungry.

To keep this simple, when your body believes that there seems to be a shortage of food, its "metabolic thermostat" begins to crank down its functions, in order for it to require less energy to run. (Essentially, it's like if you see that your income has decreased, you'd try to cut some of your expenses in order to survive. Your body does the "survival finances" for you.)

And especially NEAT - you'd notice that you'd feel more tired, you're less willing to move around, and you fidget less, etc.

But why did I say that this drop isn't really significant when it comes to fat loss? To explain this, let's take a trip back in time.

The Dark Side of Scientific Knowledge

We know that during World War II, the Nazi's kept prisoners in their concentration camps. These prisoners were kept daily on an intake of 700-800 calories. On top of such low caloric intake, they were forced to do hard labour, so their net daily calories is likely extremely little. This went on for months and months! This was a real starvation.

We know that these prisoners were most likely in a highly stressed state (of course). They probably also didn't sleep well. And they were starving every day.

They were breaking every single "rule" of conventional fat loss.

But did they stop losing weight? Did they plateau? Did they get fat?

The answers to all of those questions were, of course, **NO.**

Obviously, there were no fat prisoners. The fact was that they were in a calorie deficit. Now I'm 100% NOT saying go ahead and starve yourself, because these prisoners experienced much more severe health deterioration than just that little "fat loss" problem we're having. They were facing real survival problems.

But the fact is that, **no metabolic decrease, hormonal changes, sleep, nor stress, can stop you from losing fat, if a proper calorie deficit is in place.**

AGAIN, I'm NOT saying you should ignore health, nor that health issues can be overridden by simply a caloric reduction. I'm merely using this example to state a biological fact.

So what should you do if after a prolonged period of calorie deficit, you still don't see any further progress?

My recommendation is that if you are experiencing an apparent "plateau" (usually after 2-3 months), try the following:

1. **Slash out another 100-200 calories** of your daily intake and observe for another week;
2. **Repeat step 1 until your daily calorie intake is just way too little** (For men, below ~1400. For women, below ~1000);
3. **Eat at maintenance calories for 3-4 weeks**, depending on how you feel. (Don't worry, when you eat at maintenance calories, you won't get fat. You'll simply "hold onto" your current body for a while.)

Step 3 is so that we "reset" hormonally, and bring your body back to its optimal functioning. This will reset you psychologically as well, and you will feel much better.

After the 3-4 weeks of maintenance calories, go back on your deficit. You'll find that your fat loss progress will resume quite nicely.

Now... To the people who use "slow metabolism" as an EXCUSE for failing to lose fat...

The fact is clear. If you're in a real calorie deficit, YOU. WILL. LOSE. FAT.

It ain't your hormones. It ain't your "fat genes". It ain't insulin. It ain't processed foods. It ain't because you were "born this way." It ain't because you caught the "obesity" disease.

Obesity is the sum of the daily decisions you made on food.

You gained weight because YOU ATE TOO MANY CALORIES - accumulated over a long time!

If that's you, then I'm going to say something you might not like hearing...

You shouldn't be looking for ways to "boost metabolism". YOU NEED TO FOCUS ON CALORIE MANAGEMENT, AND EAT LESS CALORIES.

I assume you picked up this book because you're actually looking for the truth and real solutions. So if you're offended by these facts that I've stated, then you're reading the wrong book. If not, then I congratulate you thus far in this learning journey.

Chapter 13

WORDS FOR THE LADIES

Men are simpletons. But ladies, because of the fluctuations of your hormones, there might need to be some different rules to play by. This is why I have a dedicated chapter, just for you ladies.

So to my boys, you can choose to skip this chapter.

In an average menstrual cycle of 28 days, it's divided into 2 phases: 1) the follicular phase, and 2) the luteal phase, with approximately 14 days in each phase.

Marked by the first day of your period, it's the beginning of the follicular phase (let's call it "phase 1" for simplicity). Approximately 14 days after, it's when ovulation happens. Ovulation marks the beginning of the luteal phase (let's call it "phase 2" for simplicity).

So to conclude, the two most important days to note are 1) the first day of your period, and 2) the ovulation day, because they mark the end of a previous phase and the beginning of a new phase.

Why is it important to identify these phases? Because they could affect your cravings, willpower, and physical performance. Let's talk about how you'd feel in these two phases.

The Follicular Phase (Phase 1)

Although this phase begins with your period which may include physical discomfort, this phase is where you tend to feel stronger and more energetic. Here are some characteristics of this phase:

- Physically stronger
- More energetic
- Less bloating and water weight
- Less cravings

The Luteal Phase (Phase 2)

While you may feel the sexiest during ovulation, it marks the beginning of the second phase. Here are some characteristics of this phase:

- More likely to feel moody
- More cravings for higher-calorie foods
- More likelihood for bloating and water retention
- Physically weaker, but higher muscular recovery rate
- Less energetic

But the good news is, to counteract the cravings during this phase, your BMR is actually higher by approximately 7% (on average). This equates to about 100 extra calories per day.

Many women find it easier to keep things in control in phase 1, but rather a hell to deal with in phase 2. This is usually because of a lack of understanding and strategy for the two natural phases. In order to enjoyably lose fat and keep your dream physique, you need to understand your body and work with it.

Here are some tips I have for you:

1. In phase 1, you can try to be stricter with your calorie and nutritional targets. This is because during this phase, your willpower is higher and you have fewer cravings to deal with. So this is your opportunity to get focused on getting to your goals.

2. In phase 2, don't try to fight your body too hard. It's important to understand that the cravings are natural because of that higher metabolism. Your body during this phase needs a bit more energy to do what it needs to do.

3. In phase 2, listen to how your body feels. If cravings are strong, allow yourself to eat at maintenance calories +7%. If you feel that they're not too strong, and you feel fine, you may proceed with your calorie deficit.

4. Most cravings during phase 2 are foods with a combination of high fats and simple carbs (such as sugar). This is why most women during phase 2 crave chocolate. When you have these cravings, don't try to fight against it. Instead:

    a. Allocate some calories to enjoy some of those foods you crave. Yes, these could include your favourite desserts. Just make sure that you're also eating other foods that are satiating.

b. Consider swapping out some of your sweets (simple sugar) for more "starchy carbs", such as noodles, rice, pasta, wheat, potatoes, especially complex kinds (such as brown rice, sweet potatoes, whole wheat, etc.). The more you "spoil" your body with sweets, the more it understands their availability and craves them. This is important because the less you spoil your body, the more comfortable you'll actually feel.

c. Balance points A and B above.

In practice, you could plan your nutrition so that your calorie deficit only happens in phase 1, and in phase 2 you're eating up to maintenance calories (+7%), depending on how you feel.

Chapter 14

LET'S WORKOUT: EXERCISE SELECTION

To know how to design our training plan, we need to, once again, be clear with our goals. For the purpose of our book, our goal is to transform into *THE* physique we talked about in Chapter 5 - the sexy, lean, and toned celebrity-like physique.

Let's break down the male celebrity physique first.

Chris Hemsworth has arguably one of the most popularly sought physiques. At first glance, the most obvious feature is his wide shoulder-to-waist ratio, which gives his upper body that powerful look. His abs and muscle definition gives him that lean low-body-fat look. His round 3-dimensional shoulders and that evenly-developed chest give him that strong masculine appearance. Let's turn him around also, we can see that he's got that v-tapered back that's also defined due to a low body fat.

Next is Eddie Peng. Both Eddie and Chris have similar characteristics, with Eddie being a milder version. The 2 key traits are 1) wide shoulder-to-waist ratio, and 2) low body fat.

What we get from that is, we need to focus on these key areas:

1. Shoulders
2. Chest
3. V-taper characteristic of the back (Lats)
4. Mid-back
5. Low body fat

To hit those areas, we need to perform what I call **Aesthetic Compound Movements (ACM)**. In exercise science, a **Compound Movement** is a resistance training movement that requires multiple muscle groups to exert force, often allowing the performance of heavier load, and thus maximum strength gain. Here are the key ACMs for men:

1. **For shoulders: Some sort of vertically pushing movement** (such as seated dumbbell shoulder press, overhead press, or handstand push-up)
2. **For chest: Some sort of horizontally pushing movement** (such as bench press or incline chest press, depending on which part of the chest - upper or lower - an individual needs to focus on, for that evenly-developed look; or push-up)
3. **For lats: Some sort of vertically pulling movement** (such as pull-up or assisted pull-up, lat pulldown, etc.)

4. **For mid-back: Some sort of horizontally pulling movement** (such as seated row, dumbbell row, bent-over row, etc.)

"But Andy, What about abs?"

The fact is, your abs aren't a big muscle. To "have abs", 99% of it isn't from training, but rather your nutrition (by being in a calorie deficit). The key to having abs is to have your body fat be low enough to reveal them.

To have that amazing head-turning beach body six-pack abs, your body fat needs to be approximately 9-11%. Any higher, and your abs won't be as sharp. Any lower, and it becomes too defined that most people may find "gross" or "scary". (Interestingly, science has shown that women find the sweet spot of men's body fat to be somewhere in that range on average.)

Alright, let's now take a look at that physique for the ladies.

In Chapter 5, we've previously identified that physique, and Kendall Jenner and Nana represent this physique perfectly.

Perhaps their most attractive trait is the hourglass look. This look consists of 2 parts: 1) wide at the hips, 2) thin at the waist. Next, they look lean but not too lean. When abs on women look too defined, they may be crossing into that masculine look. Kendall's abdominal area has that "3-line" look, but not a full-blown six-pack. Now when they raise their arms, we can see that their upper body has some v-taper to it. This further enhances the appearance of that thin waist. From the side angle, we can see that they have some chest muscles, which give the breasts a "push-up" effect.

Now let's take a look at the lower body. They both have slim legs, making the visual appearance taller and their legs longer. This visual effect comes from her thighs not being too bulky. And damn, look at the glutes! They both have well-proportioned glutes that match the entire look of their lower bodies, and don't make them look too stocky!

Along with the "3-lined" abs, we can also see that leanness from the defined arms and legs. This is a sign of low body fat.

What we get from analyzing Kendall and Nana is, we need to focus on these key areas:

1. Glutes
2. Hip width
3. Chest
4. V-taper characteristic of the back (Lats)
5. Mid-back
6. 3-lined abs

So for women's key ACMs, they are:

1. **For glutes: Some sort of hip thrusting movement** (such as barbell hip thrust, bodyweight hip thrust, etc.)
2. **For hip width: Some sort of hip abduction movement** (such as hip abduction machine, cable hip abduction, banded hip abduction, etc.)
3. **For chest: Some sort of horizontally pushing movement** (same as men)

4. **For lats: Some sort of vertically pulling movement** (same as men)
5. **For mid-back: Some sort of horizontally pulling movement** (same as men)
6. **For 3-lined abs: Calorie deficit to achieve low body fat**

What body fat is low enough to have that 3-lined ab look? For women, that's approximately 17-19%.

FAQ: "What about squats and deadlifts? Aren't those essential compound movements?"

Let me first call BS on that.

Most people, including trainers, don't understand the purpose of squats and deadlifts. They assume EVERYONE needs to do them, because:

1. These people will somehow be "structurally weak" or lack balance of muscular strength, and fall apart, or;
2. Squats and deadlifts are "of course" key movements that apply to everything.

And both of the above are not true.

First, to assume that without squats and deadlift that'll cause problems by just strengthening other areas is just simply false. Strengthening one area does not cause an automatic weakening of another. Most people don't do any physical exercises at all, and structurally they're just fine. Why would it be the case that if they trained their chest and back, all of a sudden, their legs would fall apart? That simply doesn't make any sense.

If you actually have problems in your lower body and are required to strengthen your lower body, then this is beyond the scope of this book. You may need to seek a physiotherapist or other appropriate professionals. The goal of this book isn't to cover all aspects of life and all your problems.

Now, addressing the second point above, in NO cases in life should we apply a "cookie-cutting" assumption to anything. And this rings true for squats and deadlifts as well. There is definitely a time and place for squats and deadlifts to be done. (Personally, I incorporate them in my own training routine.) However, the purpose of the book is to build *THE* physique that we see in celebrities, that lean "sexy" beach body. **So for men, the focus is on the upper body. For women, that's the glutes, but without bulking the legs.**

So depending on your goal, squats and deadlifts may or may not be applied. The purpose of squats is usually to build size and/or ability in the legs. The purpose of deadlift is usually to build functional lifting strength. None of those apply to our goal.

Again, I'm not saying that squats and deadlifts aren't important. But remember that, especially as beginners, we have a limited ability to recover and build. We can't do everything all at once. For example, you don't see a professional soccer player doing lots of upper body training on top of their lower body performance-focused training. It's not that the upper body isn't important. It's that **they MUST focus on ONE THING at a time**.

The same principle applies here. If you want to get that physique, then we need focus on getting that physique first. When you arrive at the final physique you're after, and THEN you decide that you want explosive jumping abilities, or one-arm chin-up ability, or extreme running endurance, by all means go for it!

By the way, to those "professionals" that claim that doing squats won't build size on the legs "that easily"…

Yes. The truth is, it actually will. Even for women. Sure, it won't make your legs as thick as Arnold Schwarzenegger, but I believe that some women like to keep their legs as slim as they can to give them a "long" appearance. Doing squats would be counterproductive to that specific goal.

Always remember YOUR OWN purpose of doing something. Don't blindly do it just because someone told you this other reason is "important".

FAQ: "I don't want to get too big. I just want to be more toned. Should I also do these exercises?"

This **IS** the way to get toned. We must not underestimate the amount of lean mass a "toned" person has. To have muscular tone, you first need… well… muscles!

To explain what being "toned" is, let's simplify our body into a general concept of a 3-layered cylinder.

The innermost layer is our bones and skeleton. Nothing we need to do there, as that's determined by genetics. The middle layer is our lean mass (muscles). Finally, the outermost layer is our fat mass, covering everything.

To look toned, you must increase the middle layer (muscles) slightly, and drastically thin out the outermost layer of fat. When the outermost layer of fat is thin, your body will take on the shape of the dense middle layer, giving your body a lean toned look.

If you trained for size for years and years (I'm talking at least 3-5 years) of proper weightlifting, then you'll get "bigger". But muscle growth is an extremely slow process. So trust me, you won't wake up one morning, surprised to find yourself to have grown past your "ideal" size. You'll have plenty of time to control what size you're happy with.

Now that we've broken down the key training areas we need, let's go onto some more specifics as to how we should train ourselves.

Chapter 15

THE MAIN PRINCIPLE OF TRAINING

There is a major flaw in the fitness industry. It's why most fitness regimes and group classes don't deliver the results you're looking for. You may lose a few pounds and gain some muscles at first, but then you'd notice that nothing changes further from there.

Why?

Because they all lack the one single main principle of all training.

It's called **Progressive Overload**.

Progressive overload is simply training with an increased resistance or difficulty, in order to challenge your body's progressive adaptation to the previous resistance or difficulty.

In other words, your training needs to be progressively getting harder!

Without progressive overload, there is no reason for your body to change! Upon introduction of a "new stimulus" (your training) to your body, the resistance "breaks down" your muscles, to the extent of the difficulty relative to your body's capability. After the training, your body repairs itself, but... not only does it recover back to where it was, it "remembers" that difficult stimulus you introduced earlier, and "adapts" by building MORE muscle fibres than you've previously had. Because of that procedure, its capability will increase, and a new "normal" would be set.

In exercise science, we call that **"supercompensation"**. (Refer to Chapter 16, Priority 6 for more detail.)

Later on, if stimuli of similar difficulty (compared to your "normal") were introduced, your body wouldn't need to adapt again. And until a more difficult resistance is introduced, your body will more or less stay the same.

Now, going back to what you would regularly see in the fitness industry... Do you see the problem here?

Most fitness classes (especially group training) don't deliver results because there are no ways for 1 instructor to take care of 30-40 people. And for regular folks, most do not understand the concept of progressive overload. They naively believe that as long as they're exercising and moving around in a fitness setting, they'll get results. Therefore, most people tend to do the same things week after week, month after month. It's no wonder that the most amazing transformation into that sexy, lean, toned beach body doesn't happen for most people.

A somewhat knowledgeable personal trainer would implement the concept of progressive overload into the backbone of your workout plans.

A training regime without progressive overload shouldn't even be called "training". That'd just be... moving around. Training regimes should serve greater purposes.

In resistance training, that progressive overload would generally be applied to strength. This is because strength is the backbone of muscle building. In other words, if your strength is incredible, your physique won't be too shabby.

This is the number one foundation in fitness. If I have to ignore everything else and pinpoint the one key factor in training to make it an effective one, it's progressive overload.

Now, let me give you an example of what progressive overload looks like in a trainee's workout log:

Mr. Lean's Dumbbell Shoulder Press
6/6: 40 lbs for 8, 7, 6 reps
6/9: 40 lbs for 9, 8, 8 reps
6/13: 40 lbs for 10, 9, 9 reps
6/15: 45 lbs for 6; 40 lbs for 9, 8 reps
6/18: 45 lbs for 7, 6; 40 lbs for 9 reps

...

10/10: 65 lbs for 7, 6; 50 lbs for 10, 10 reps

As we can see, Mr. Lean has been progressively pushing himself to do more reps, and eventually a heavier load. By October, he not only got stronger, but he was able to train with more sets. This is progressive overload.

Now that we understand the necessity of progressive overload, let's go onto how we design our workouts.

Chapter 16

TRAINING PRIORITIES

In the previous chapter, I talked about the key principle of any training. But now, before we begin planning your training, you first need to understand the priorities. This is because without understanding priorities, there's just too much noise out there.

"Keep the heart rate high and rest short between sets". Or "Take longer rest periods to ensure quality."

"Perform each rep slowly." Or "Lift fast and explosively."

"Lift heavy in low rep range." Or "Lift light and more reps."

"Focus on a few exercises." Or "Switch things up, you gotta do a wide range of exercises."

"Exercise in absolute proper form." Or "Sacrificing some form is preferred."

The problem is, these can be contradicting. So, who should you listen to?

The truth is, there's a time and place for all of those statements to be of higher priority. For example, strength training for a well-proportioned toned body is very different from condition training for athletic performance in basketball.

However, for the purpose of us getting in shape, getting to that dream celebrity-like physique, some of these factors will take on a higher priority than others.

So in this book, I'll clarify once and for all what you need to focus on, and what you don't need to worry too much about.

Here is the general ladder of priorities:

1. Exercise selection
2. Proper forms
3. Range of motion
4. Strength adaptation (with progressive overload)
5. Lifting tempo
6. Volume and recovery (with progressive overload)
7. Training frequency

Less important:

8. Mind-muscle connection
9. Rest time in between sets

Like I talked about in Chapter 5, to build *THE* physique we're after, combining with low body fat, we must build lean mass in the "right" places to ensure good proportions. To get down to low body fat, we know that the only way to get there is to have a calorie deficit in place. Previously, we talked about how too much intense cardio could be counterproductive, and we know that "spot reduction" of fat cannot be done through training. (More details about cardio in Chapter 19.)

Therefore, the primary goal of training is to build lean mass in proportion. Keep in mind, that's our goal with training (to add lean mass, NOT subtract fat mass). Now let's begin.

Priority 1: Exercise Selection

Exercise selection is the first priority. I think this is self-explanatory. If your goal is to have a wider back like Chris Hemsworth, but all you do is jogging, then that obviously wouldn't make sense. As I've talked about in Chapter 15, the details in how to select your exercises were mentioned there.

Priority 2: Proper Forms

Having proper form in the beginning stages is crucial.
A) It allows you to train the muscles intended to be trained, and
B) it can prevent you from physical injuries, some of which could be permanent.

There will be situations in more advanced lifting where strength adaptation will be higher in priority than having proper form. But for beginners, proper form is extremely important.

Priority 3: Range of Motion

During the beginner phases, range of motion is extremely important in that maximizing it can ensure your muscles being trained in all "lengths" of muscular contraction. This is key in building foundations for good muscle growth.

If you can't perform in an optimal range of motion (and it's not because of physical limitations such as injury or bone structure), you must reduce resistance or difficulty of the exercise, to ensure you can maximize the range of motion.

For example, if you can't perform a push-up all the way down (chest touching the floor) and all the way up, then kneel down to train push-ups, or do incline push-ups where your hands are situated at an elevated height. Altering ranges of motion is an advanced technique used appropriately in very specific situations, but for us, **DO NOT sacrifice range of motion** just to do a harder exercise or with a heavier load.

Priority 4: Strength Adaptation

The most important key as a stimulus for lean mass growth is progressive overload in strength. Our body doesn't care about us "looking good". The reason why we grow muscle is simply that there's a physical demand that our body can't currently perform with ease. Remember, our body is a survival machine. It changes only when it has to, not because it wants to.

To train for strength, you have to lift heavy. After all, to get stronger, you must introduce a stimulus that needs you to use your absolute strength.

If you've never had proper weight-lifting training, you shouldn't go all out lifting heavy. This is because if your body hasn't had enough time to adapt to proper lifting, lifting heavy suddenly may cause injury. And your body is too new to all this, so sudden heavy lifting isn't something that'll effectively stimulate muscle growth. Later in the book, I'll give you example routines if you're an absolute beginner.

But after building that foundation for proper lifting techniques, you want to begin lifting those key compound movements in a lower rep range (approximately 6-9 reps per set), while the resistance should be heavier - heavy enough so that your best effort would land in between that rep range. I'll give you more detailed instructions later in the book.

Priority 5: Lifting Tempo

Lifting tempo ensures muscular control and proper strength development. You don't want to be "going through the motion" and "letting gravity do the work". Your job is to control the weight, or at least do your best to.

A general rule of thumb is to take 2 seconds on each half of the range of motion. For example, when doing a push-up, you want to take 2 seconds down, then 2 seconds up.

When the exercise is mastered in terms of form and control (usually after 2-3 weeks of consistent training), then we'll change up the tempo here. For the "concentric" part (going against gravity) of the range, you can explode the motion (as fast as you can). For the "eccentric" part (going towards gravity) you should still take 2 seconds in a controlled fashion.

For example, for the push-up, you'd explode when pushing up, then control the motion over 2 seconds when going down.

*Tip: After 2 months of consistent proper training, I suggest that for the **last rep** of all your **heavy ACM sets**, perform the **eccentric part extremely slowly, taking 6-8 seconds**.*

Priority 6: Volume and Recovery

Given the top 2 priorities (the right exercise selection, the right intensity) in place, the increase in volume is shown by science to be proportional to lean mass growth.

Volume is essentially the total "work" you've done in your workout. In simple terms:

Volume = reps x sets

However, volume (along with intensity) comes hand in hand with recovery. If you can't recover, that's when more volume won't build more muscles. A proper stimulus to start muscle growth is one thing, but full recovery is what your body needs to actually build the muscles.

Here's a graph to show you the entire concept:

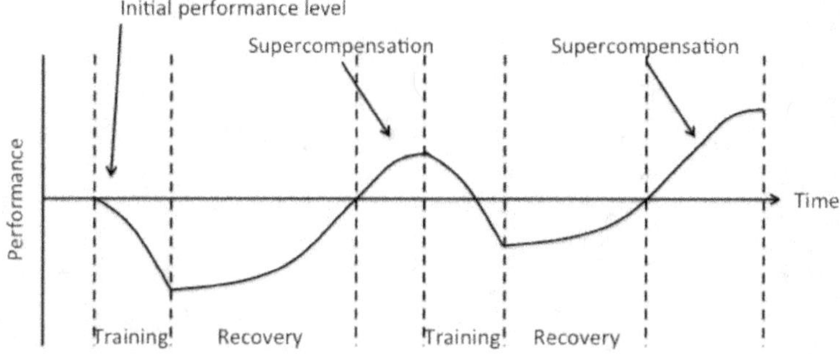

When you do a workout, depending on what the intensity and volume was, your muscles will "break down" to a certain extent, calling your body to repair. If the repair was within your body's ability, it not only repairs but also builds more muscles. This is called **supercompensation**. This is what will actually make a difference in your physique.

If you accumulate workouts after workouts without your body being able to recover, this could eventually lead to "**overtraining**". Your body's recovery cannot catch up to the extent of muscle breakdown caused by your training sessions, and this "debt" accumulates. So eventually, instead of getting stronger, you may not see any progress, or sometimes even a decrease in performance.

Here's an illustration to show you the difference:

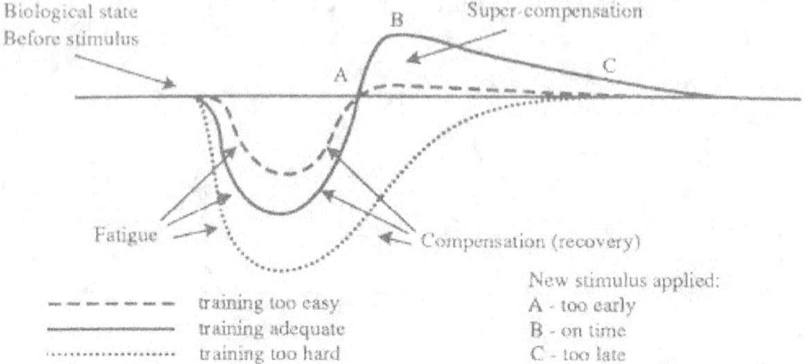

As I mentioned before, your willpower battery would also take a hit if your body is unable to recover, causing an accumulation of fatigue. So obviously, we don't want that.

Here, I should mention that, even if you properly trained at the optimal volume, your body may still decrease in its ability to recover eventually, as you train consistently and the days go by. So gradually, even with proper training and optimal volume, you'll reach a point of fatigue regardless. This is completely normal, and you aren't doing anything wrong. We just want to make sure that you were training at your optimal volume in the first place, to prevent overtraining from happening too soon.

Long story short, you need to choose the perfect volume for you, in order to maximize muscle-building speed. As mentioned before, the muscle-building process is an extremely slow one, so effective training is very important, in order to look good.

Priority 7: Training Frequency

Training frequency is the next priority. Not as high up as the others, but if done, this could make an easy difference in your results.

Science has shown that, given all the above priorities in place (same intensity, same volume, etc.), when you compare the total weekly workout volume split into 2 days per week, with the same volume but split into 4 days, even though throughout the week you're doing the same amount of "work", the 4-day split produces better lean mass gains!

This means, you can have shorter training times per session, as long as you train a bit more often.

It's strongly recommended that you train **each muscle group twice per week**.

So overall, I recommend your training frequency to be **4 days per week** for optimal growth. But you should try to design your routine at a frequency of at least 2 days per week.

Below is my recommendation for how you should split your routine.

For Men

Training Frequency Per Week	Day 1	Day 2	Day 3	Day 4
2	Full-body	Full-body		
3	Push	Pull	Full-body	
4	Push	Pull	Push	Pull

Training Frequency Per Week	Day 1	Day 2	Day 3	Day 4
2	Full-body	Full-body		
3	Lower	Upper	Full-body	
4	Lower	Upper	Lower	Upper

Now having said that, DON'T BE A PERFECTIONIST. This comes down to how available you are to go to the gym. If you're not able to go to the gym frequently, remember that as long as your other "higher-up" priorities are in place, you'll still get most of the results! So don't let frequency be an excuse for you to quit. Training at lower frequency is still WAY better than none at all.

I'll provide some sample workout routines you can use later in the book.

Less Important Factor 1: Mind-Muscle Connection

As a beginner, this aspect is less important. Many trainers overemphasize the importance of mind-muscle connection.

But the fact is that, when you're a beginner, your muscles aren't optimized to "feel" much. Your nervous system hasn't developed enough "muscle recruitment" abilities. In other words, you're too inexperienced to feel the muscles, until you practice more and get stronger.

Many beginners wonder why even though a push-up is considered a "chest" exercise, but after the workout they "feel it in their arms more". That's the reason. They're simply not strong enough.

However, you may have seen many advanced trainees being able to contract their muscles at will, such as seeing a muscular guy "bouncing" his chest muscles. The reason he can do that is that he has the ability to recruit chest muscle fibres easily due to training experience.

Mind-muscle connection certainly has a place in training, and it will come into play after a few weeks or months of proper training. But not right at the beginning. In the beginning, you should worry more about having actual proper form, instead of "feeling" out what's right.

That being said, there's a time and place for mind-muscle connection to be implemented. Its main implementation is during isolation exercises, which are usually not done in the beginning.

Less Important Factor 2: Rest Times in Between Sets

Most people, even fitness "professionals" and influencers, believe it's important to "keep the heart rate high" by reducing rest time. But if your goal is to build *THE* physique as we talked about in the book, then rest time isn't that important. In fact, you should keep the rest time slightly higher (especially for compound movements).

Some people may bring up the argument, *"but Andy, by keeping the heart rate high, you'd burn more calories, which helps with fat loss and toning."*

As I talked about in Chapter 15, toning means 1) thin out the body fat layer, and 2) slightly enlarge the muscle layer.

While it's true that keeping the heart rate high will cause you to burn more calories, it's not always true that it will definitely "help" with fat loss.

First, even if you kept the heart rate high, you won't be burning THAT many more calories anyway. We're talking about around 50-100 calories extra. That's not that much, and certainly can't be relied on for fat loss.

Second, fat loss comes from an OVERALL calorie deficit, which means that even if you burned a lot of calories during a workout, if your bodily signals made you eat more later on, and it ruined that calorie deficit, you still won't lose fat. (I talked about this point in detail earlier in the book.) Plus, that extra 50-100 calories can EASILY be eaten. And all that hard work doesn't translate to more calories, but instead, leaves you hungry for more.

So instead, the "thinning out body fat" part should come primarily from your diet creating that calorie deficit, while training should be focused on building that muscle layer (in the right "good-looking" ratio). Combining the two, this will ultimately produce that dream body.

So you should actually rest longer between sets is that strength and volume progressive overload (as we talked about earlier is the key to building muscle) relies on QUALITY lifting heavy loads, as science has shown over and over again. That means, you'd rather rest longer to ensure the quality of next sets, rather than "keeping heart rate high" but half-assing later sets due to fatigue.

(See Chapter 19 for more details on cardio or cardio-like exercises.)

Now that you have the priorities in mind for what an effective training system should look like, let's go on to give you some examples.

Chapter 17

YOUR TRAINING ROUTINE

The following examples I'm going to give you are general, and for beginners only. It'd be impossible for me to give you examples for everyone, because everyone is different.

Let's start with the ladies.

So for women's key ACMs, they are:
1.   For glutes: Hip thrust
2.   For hip width: Hip abduction
3.   For lower chest: Incline push-up
4.   For lats: Lat pulldown or assisted pull-up machine
5.   For mid-back: Wide-grip seated row

To optimize results, we should increase the frequency to hitting each muscle group 2 times per week. And do so by going to the gym 4 times (2 days of upper body training, 2 days of lower). So for an **absolute beginner**, it'd look something like this:

Day 1 - Lower Body

- Lower body warm-up routine
- Hip thrust (Barbell, smith machine, or dumbbell): 3 sets of 10-15 reps, 2-minute rest per set
- Hip abduction machine: 3 sets of 10-15 reps, 1.5-minute rest per set
- (Add in 1 month later) Straight-legged cable kickback: 2 sets of 15-20 reps, 1-minute rest per set

Day 2 - Upper Body

- Upper body warm-up routine
- Incline push-up: 2 sets of 10-15 reps, 2-minute rest per set
- Lat pulldown: 2 sets of 10-15 reps, 2-minute rest per set
- Wide-grip seated row: 2 sets of 10-15 reps, 2-minute rest per set
- (Add in 1 month later) Dumbbell lateral raise: 2 sets of 10-15 reps, 1.5-minute rest per set

NOTES:

1. Warm-up routines are essential. The purposes are A) prevent injury, B) activate muscles intended to be used for more strength during a workout, and better results from the workout.
2. Use light weight so that you can comfortably perform the exercise in the rep ranges indicated. Focus more on proper form and control, rather than lifting heavy and "muscle feel".

3. Although some women don't like having big thighs and legs, the squat could be a functional exercise to ensure strong healthy legs. Performing 2 sets is sufficient for that, if that's what you want. However, refer to the FAQ in Chapter 14 when deciding if squats is something you need to do.

After 2-3 weeks when you've mastered the form and control of these exercises, you should:

1. Decrease the target rep range to 8-12 reps for ACMs (and squats).
2. Decrease the target rep range to 10-15 reps for movements other than ACMs (and squats).
3. Choose a weight that you can perform with maximum effort and land in that rep range above.
4. Increase the number of sets per exercise to 3.
5. Increase the rest time to 3 minutes for ACMs if needed.
6. Keep up the "progressive overload" to ensure that, with maximum effort, you're landing in that rep range above. This means, if you're hitting closer to the top end of the rep range, make a note that you can try a heavier load next time. (For example, if you can do a 30-lb lat pulldown for 12 reps, then next time, you should want to try 40 lbs.)

Now, onto the gentlemen.

Day 1 - Push

- Upper Body warm-up routine
- Seated dumbbell shoulder press, 2 sets of 10-15 reps, 2-minute rest per set
- Incline dumbbell chest press, 2 sets of 10-15 reps, 2-minute rest per set
- Dumbbell tricep extension, 2 sets of 10-15 reps, 1.5-minute rest per set
- (Add in 1 month later) Dumbbell lateral raise, 2 set of 10-15 reps, 1.5-minute rest per set

Day 2 - Pull

- Upper body warm-up routine
- Lat pulldown: 2 sets of 10-15 reps, 2-minute rest per set
- Wide-grip seated row: 2 sets of 10-15 reps, 2-minute rest per set
- Standing dumbbell bicep curl: 2 sets of 10-15 reps, 1.5-minute rest per set
- (Add in 1 month later) Machine pec deck: 2 sets of 10-15 reps, 1.5-minute rest per set

NOTES:

1. Warm-up routines are essential. The purposes are A) prevent injury, B) activate muscles intended to be used for more strength during a workout, and better results from the workout.

2. Use light weight so that you can comfortably perform the exercise in the rep ranges indicated. Focus more on proper form and control, rather than lifting heavy and "muscle feel".

After 2-3 weeks when you've mastered the form and control of these exercises, you should:

1. Decrease the target rep range to 7-10 reps for ACMs.
2. Choose a weight that you can perform with maximum effort and land in that rep range above.
3. Increase the number of sets per exercise to 3.
4. Increase the rest time to 3 minutes for ACMs if needed.
5. Keep up the "progressive overload" to ensure that, with maximum effort, you're landing in that rep range above. This means, if you're hitting closer to the top end of the rep range, make a note that you can try a heavier load next time. (For example, if you can do a 30-lb lat pulldown for 12 reps, then next time, you should want to try 40 lbs.)

NOTE: The volume for this routine works for the frequency of 4 training days per week. If you're training at a lower frequency (such as 2-3 days per week), you'd need to **increase the volume per workout session slightly**.

Remember your lifting tempo, which is extremely important in getting real results. Refer to Chapter 16, Priority 5.

FAQ: "Why use mostly dumbbells? What about barbells?"

When you first start training, dumbbells would be the better choice for two big reasons:

1. **You train your muscles to be able to control free weights.**

   o There are small muscles in your body called "stabilizer muscles". It's important to train them along the way so you don't lag behind in the future due to having weak stabilizers.

   o Imagine you trained with only machines since the beginning (zero stabilizer training). After a year, in order to progress further, you go to barbells. But because you have weak stabilizers, you're unable to lift the same weight with a barbell as the weight you used with machines. To fix this, you'd have to go back down in weight, and "re-train" your way back up. That'd suck, right?

2. **Everyone has a dominant side, which can cause an imbalance in muscle growth if not separately trained.**

   o If you went directly into barbells right from the start, chances are, you will lift the barbell with your dominant side contributing to the motion more than your weaker side.

   o This causes your dominant side to be trained consistently more than the weaker side, causing the gap between the two sides to become increasingly bigger.

- o An important part of aesthetics is having physical symmetry. I think most people wouldn't want one side to be way bigger than the other.

FAQ: "Only 3-4 exercises? Are you sure this would be effective?"

Many people, including many trainers, overestimate the complexity of building a good physique. Right when they begin their fitness journey, they perform lots and lots of different exercises.

The fact is that, as an intermediate or advanced trainee, you'll most likely need a lot more exercises to further build the physique you're after. But **as a beginner**, your ability to recover is limited - so you need to focus all your limited bodily ability on building that "structural foundation", which is the underlying key to any great physique. **And such foundation comes from progressive overload in the ACMs**.

The fact is, **ACMs will produce 90% of your physical results.** The rest are just "finishing touches" that won't make a real difference unless your foundation strengths are there. Literally, if you just make sure you improve in your ACM performance, you can already build a body that's more aesthetic than your average gym-goers.

Over the period of time that my girlfriend learned about physique transformation from me, she's greatly transformed her physique into one that she's very satisfied with (for now). And from her transformation, this is how she describes the training aspect.

She felt that the entire training journey is like completing an advanced painting. As a painter, you probably wouldn't go straight into putting the paint right on the canvas. You'd need to use a pencil, and probably roughly draw out the basic structural foundation of the final product.

Training is the same. The initial months of proper training focuses on building that "structural" foundation. By doing lots and lots of different exercises, there'd be no focus. The end result of that would be "messy", with no real transformation seen. Your training and result would be like a "jack of all trades", but "master of none".

And she's tried that way previously, and gotten no visible results.

But when she focused her workouts around the few key ACMs, within a few months, she saw significant body changes. And the changes in the key body parts that she'd find attractive (such as the gluteus and the back) became very prominent.

Just like a painting, focus on the foundations first. Everything else would just be used as "finishing touches".

FAQ: "Why are the workouts so short? I didn't even sweat."

Most people overestimate how much exercise it takes to build a good physique. In fact, there is a "just right Goldilocks" principle for the amount of training volume you need. More isn't always more.

There are two reasons you need to consider. First, as a beginner, you don't need that much volume to "tell your body" you need to grow muscle. Second, as a beginner, you don't have that much capability to recover. As mentioned in the previous chapter, too much volume can actually stall you from progressing.

Next, sweating is NOT a good indicator of an effective workout. Sweating is simply a result of your body heating up, which has nothing to do with muscle stimulation and growth.

Remember, we're not trying to burn calories from the workout because of the reasons I mentioned earlier in the book. So we must remember why we're training in the first place: to build lean mass in the right area, so that combining with a calorie deficit, we can achieve that toning effect and build "that" physique we're after.

As You Progress...

As you progress through proper training, you should notice a significant strength and muscle gain in just a few months or even weeks! Pat yourself on the back for the good work! You can begin to push the strength of ACMs more and more...

But I strongly don't suggest increasing the number of sets of ACMs to more than 4 sets per exercise, as usually performing 3 sets is more than enough to stimulate good muscle growth for a long while.

For the isolation exercises (such as lateral raise, pec deck, tricep push down, etc.), you don't need it until after 2-3 months of proper training. After that, you may begin to add a few sets of those to further increase volume and sculpt your body. However…

EXTREMELY IMPORTANT: Do so extremely carefully and UNDER ONE CONDITION ONLY: Your main ACMs must be continuing to progress.

The progressive overload of our ACMs is our MAIN goal. If that's jeopardized, it doesn't matter how crazy the amounts of sets and reps you do, **YOUR PHYSIQUE WON'T IMPROVE!**

I can't stress this point enough, as most people think "more is better", and they keep piling on more and more sets (some people do 10 or 20 sets of the same exercise in one go). These meatheads always say "no pain no gain" or "go hard or go home", and they may sound all cool and inspiring, but it's just dumb and not scientific at all.

And for others, they may appear to have hit a "plateau" in their strength or physique gains, and they think they need to "break through" their plateaus by adding more sets. And they usually end up not gaining more, and often they lose their strength.

Why? Because more volume means they cannot recover. And recovery is when your body builds muscles, NOT when you're actually training. So NO. The answer isn't more sets. The answer is often LESS volume.

I've talked about the concept of overtraining vs. overreaching. So if you need a review, go back to Chapter 16, under "Volume and Recovery".

<u>General Rule of Thumb</u>: **If the strength in your ACMs is progressing just fine, DO NOT change your workout formula. In general, you DO NOT need more than 4 sets for ACM (of approximately 6-10 reps) per exercise per workout.**

You may choose to increase your volume for isolation exercises as you go, but you DO NOT need more than 5 sets (of approximately 10-20 reps) per exercise per workout. If you find that, by increasing your volume, your strength in your ACMs actually slowed down or is stalled completely, then you need to go back to the volume that was working for you earlier.

So remember, it's not always "the more the better".

By the way, for isolation exercises, you can start to incorporate slower tempos and the "mind-muscle connection" approach.

FAQ: "From doing the workouts you've suggested, initially I felt sore a day or two after doing it. But after a week or two, I don't feel sore anymore. Are you sure your workouts are effective? Should I be doing something else?"

Here's a typical logic of "The existence of A always means B. But if A doesn't exist, it doesn't always mean B doesn't exist."

Here. Let me put this in regular folks' language.

If your body feels sore, it definitely means the workout was effective to some degree. BUT if your body doesn't feel sore, it doesn't always mean it wasn't effective.

This soreness that you experience is called "delayed-onset muscle soreness" (DOMS). It occurs generally for two reasons:

1. You're working out in a new way, or you haven't done your workout in a long time, OR;

2. You've progressively overloaded the eccentric part of certain movements (see Chapter 16 for what "eccentric" means).

Although those 2 above generally means it was an effective workout, an effective workout isn't JUST defined by those 2 things.

In our pursuit of that generally-liked lean beach body, part of that goal is to build lean muscle in the right proportions. And as we talked about before, that mainly comes from **progressive overload** in strength in an appropriate training volume.

That means, if:

1. You're seeing improvements (especially strength) in your workout;

2. You see numerical differences (such as number of reps, the weight you're using, or body fat, body weight, waist circumference, etc.), and;

3. You literally see physique improvements in the mirror or photos.

These 3 things above are way more important to indicate that you have an effective training regime in place, rather than just feeling whether or not you're sore after your workouts.

FAQ: *"How come the strengths of my ACMs aren't improving anymore?"*

This happens because of 3 possible reasons:

1. You aren't giving your workout your best. Yes, you should be resting longer in between sets, but when you do hit each set, you need to give it all you got, 100% effort. You can't hold back. **If this is the reason, fix this first before moving onto the next 2 points.**

2. If point 1 isn't the problem, and you still NEVER really see much strength gains, then your training volume is way too high. That means you're doing too many sets. Reduce the number of sets (especially for isolation movements) by 1 and observe what happens. Remember, if your training volume is too high for you, you're either overreaching without adaptation, or you're heading towards overtraining - neither of these cases is good. But...

3. If you saw good strength gains for a while (for at least 3-6 months), but now you're no longer improving (and I mean, not improving AT ALL with at least 1 month of consistent training, or even a decrease in strength), then you probably also feel somewhat fatigued. If that's the case, read the next FAQ.

FAQ: "I've been feeling fatigued. It's like I can't focus during my workout. It's not that I'm tired and don't have energy per se, it's more like a mental type of fatigue. I'm trying to give it my all, but my strength level seems to have plateaued as well. What should I do?"

If this is what you're experiencing, then I got a question for you.

- **If you're a beginner (0-12 months of proper training):** Have you been consistently training for at least 6 months now?

- **If you've been properly training (my way) for at least 12 months:** Have you been consistently training for at least 3 months now?

If your answer is yes, then...

Step 1) You need to reduce the volume of your workouts by 1 set for each exercise, especially ACMs.

Then observe for 2 weeks and see your energy level. If it improves, then this is your new workout volume, and you'll continue to do this volume. This means your previous training volume was too high and your body was unable to recover. You could try to increase volume later on (in a few months), but you increased volume too prematurely, and you shouldn't do that now. But if things did not improve after volume reduction, then go onto the next step.

Step 2) You need to take a "de-load week".

You're only going to do 2 sets of your ACMs on your workout days, and only at 50% of both volume and resistance. During your de-load week, also eat at maintenance calories. Do not eat at a deficit!

The reason why you need a de-load week is that we've eliminated the possibility that you're fatigued due to the inability to recover from high volume training. If you still couldn't recover even after a volume reduction, then it means your body truly burnt out from a prolonged period of proper training, and you need a break. This "de-load" is like an active rest.

So remember, as I talked about in Chapter 16, even if you properly trained at the optimal volume, your body's ability to recover will decrease, as you train consistently and the days go by. This is completely normal, and you haven't done anything wrong. You just now need a de-load break.

For the Ladies

As I mentioned earlier, in "phase 2", you probably won't be at your maximum energy. During this time, if you feel like you can't perform as heavy or difficult as when you were in phase 1, LADIES, LADIES, LADIES... you must drop the ego, and go lighter! Just remember, your monthly cycles are natural, it's okay! You'll still make excellent progress, I promise. Don't ever beat yourself up over it!

During phase 2, you may decrease intensity. But in phase 1, it's your strong time! Use the opportunity of phase 1 to push for more progressive overloading!

Patience

1   Muscle Building

The muscle-building process is actually an extremely slow one by nature. If you're trying to build more lean mass, and you wonder why you're not really gaining much weight, DO NOT eat in a huge surplus.

This is because your body has limited abilities to build muscles (unless you're taking drugs). In the first whole year, you're looking at only 10-20 lbs of muscle (depending on your genetics, height, and how efficient your training is). And for women, that's even less.

Imagine you have a factory, and its workforce is limited to 10 people. They all have a limited speed at which they work. The best you can do is to give it just enough work so that they get the most done. Just because you give them more work, doesn't mean your factory will get more done. Because the working speed by nature is limited, the work will just pile up.

Your body is the same. Just because you give it more calories, doesn't mean it's fast enough to convert them all into muscles. The excess calories will simply be stored as body fat, which is counterproductive if you're trying to go for that lean toned look.

2   Fat Loss

Fat loss is also a patience game. Your body has a limited speed in burning fat as well. The maximum efficiency in fat loss comes from a 30% calorie deficit if your body fat is in the "high" tier (as mentioned in Chapter 12). And that efficiency decreases to around 20% as your body fat gets lower, and 10-15% as your body becomes even leaner.

If you create a deficit bigger than that maximum your body can handle, your body won't actually burn more fat. Instead, because of its limited speed in burning fat, AND your impatient demand as a result of the bigger deficit you created, it will cut into your muscle mass for that extra energy. So essentially, you'd be losing muscle for no good reason, and that's just pointless.

Bottom line is, BE PATIENT. I've given you the ways with the MAXIMUM efficiency already. So please, if you want to save the trouble of failing, don't try to "speed" up muscle building or fat loss.

Chapter 18

CARDIO: DO'S AND DON'TS

There are just way too many BS out there in terms of cardio that it definitely deserves a chapter on its own. Here, I'm going to summarize all the myths, truths, the do's and don'ts.

Concept 1: The idea that "cardio directly causes you to lose fat" is FALSE.

Cardio doesn't burn fat "by itself" magically. It needs to be taken into the big picture of total net calories to determine whether or not you're "burning fat". Any form of cardio, just like any physical movements in general, is simply "negative calories" when accounting for your overall net calories.

For your body to be in a "fat burning state", it's simply as a **result of a negative net energy balance**. In every second of your life, your body is constantly being influenced by energy coming in and energy going out. You may be doing exercises that burn calories "out" of your body, but somewhere else in your body, it could also be breaking down the food you ate 3 hours ago and trying to store the calories coming "in" as body fat. Therefore, we can't just look at cardio as a separate event, and simply view it as something that directly causes fat loss.

No ONE single exercise can directly cause fat loss, and no ONE single type of food can directly cause fat gain.

So, if you're in a calorie deficit, that deficit balance will cause your body to make the "executive" decision to withdraw energy from your body fat.

Therefore, you can see that fat burning is governed by a larger force, and it's not localized. In other words, physically moving a body part does not cause your body to "burn fat" in that body part. It has to go through a higher-level decision, which is your overall energy balance control centre. Cardio is simply something that's at a "lower-level". It by itself doesn't directly decide whether you're going to "burn fat".

Let me give you an example. Let's say you're a big corporation, with 20 products that you sell. And each product has its own department.

Here's the issue. You hear that one of the 20 departments that they're not selling well, and its net profit within that single department is negative.

Now, as a corporation, are you going to directly begin seeking financial support from external sources (such as loans, cash injections, investors, etc.) immediately just because one product isn't selling well?

OR... Would it make more sense to first look at your 19 other product departments to see if your OVERALL net profit is a positive or negative number, before you make any big decisions?

Yes. Cardio is like that one product. And your body's decision to burn fat is like an executive decision from the board of directors in that corporation. Your body is extremely smart and efficient.

So cardio COULD potentially contribute to burning energy. But it doesn't burn fat, nor does it necessarily mean that by doing cardio you will for sure burn fat.

As well, we have the hormonal effects of cardio, which can further affect the outcome of weight change. I'll talk about this in the next concept below.

Concept 2: Consider your "return on effort investment" when doing cardio.

Your body is a survival machine. That means two things. One, it's good at storing fat for more energy, in case of food shortage. Two, it's efficient at using energy when you do any physical movements, in order to conserve energy (It's like that ECO mode in your car).

So the harsh truth is, you will often spend a lot of effort, to burn very little calories (not proportional to the amount of effort you put out).

For example, if you ran for 15 minutes at an average pace, you'd burn about 150-250 calories, depending on how big or small of a person you are. Keep in mind, 15 minutes is already a lot for the average person! If you don't believe me, try it yourself. Most people don't even have the stamina for 10 minutes of CONSTANT running.

Let's take the average of the calories burnt, that's about 200 calories. Well, what does that give you? That's about a very small bowl of rice. Or a third of a slice of cheesecake (Yes... Not even a full slice). Or half of a standard McDonald's double cheeseburger. Or half of a small-sized fries. Or 1 donut.

The point is, **IT'S NOT MUCH FOOD.**

You spend so much effort doing cardio (going hardcore, and more than you can handle), yet in return, you don't even get that much more food. That's the fact.

Oh yeah, don't forget. You can't just do this for one day, because fat loss doesn't happen over one day. You must do this EVERY day, if your fat loss strategy is simply cardio.

Yeah... that doesn't sound too practical now, does it?

Let's talk science quickly. Two main hormones will be affected when you invest too much effort into a cardio that won't give you back many calories.

Hormone 1 - Leptin

Leptin is the satiation hormone, which means you want to keep it high for any food you eat to feel satiating. When leptin is low, you'll start to feel like no matter how much food you eat, you're still hungry. And leptin begins to drop more significantly as you 1) are in a significant calorie deficit (usually greater than 800 cal), and 2) do cardio sessions that are at least moderately intense (around 60% of your max heart rate).

Hormone 2 - Cortisol

Cortisol is the stress hormone. In general, it increases the more intense your cardio session is, and the greater calorie deficit you're in. As well, if you're using willpower to do something (in this case, if you dislike the cardio session), cortisol can also rise. Now here's the down side. Cortisol can also cause you to eat. So as you can see here, more cardio doesn't always mean successful fat loss.

In the end, cardio is a double-edged sword. It's not as simple as "more cardio, more fat loss".

Concept 3: The "afterburn effect of HIIT cardio isn't actually that much.

Many people think that HIIT cardio is the way to go for fat loss, because of that "afterburn effect". And even a lot of fitness centres market this idea to attract more uninformed customers.

What is the afterburn effect really?

The afterburn effect, scientifically known as excess post-exercise oxygen consumption (EPOC), means that your body uses up energy (calories) to recover from a high-intensity cardio exercise. This happens when high-intensity cardio puts your body into a high-heart-rate state, your body goes into an oxygen "debt". Your body uses oxygen so rapidly during HIIT, it becomes unable to recover the oxygen your body fully needs.

So yes, while it's true that your body will need to use up energy to recover, which means that even if you're not physically doing anything after the HIIT session, you're still burning calories... The real question is...

How many calories exactly is the afterburn effect really burning for you?

Science has shown that the afterburn effect is about 6-15% (averaging to be about 10%) of your total calories burned by the HIIT session.

Let's put that into perspective. The average person burns about 300 calories from a HIIT cardio session. But let's just say this person worked really hard and managed to burn 500 calories...

Well. That's still just 50 calories from the afterburn effect. This amount of calories is so little that it doesn't make any difference in helping you create and staying in that calorie deficit.

So the take-home message here is: don't do HIIT cardio for the single reason of chasing the afterburn effect, just to lose fat. It's not worth your effort if you don't love it.

My Recommendations for Cardio

- The number one criterion for my cardio recommendation is that you MUST enjoy it. DO NOT do a cardiovascular activity PURELY for fat loss.
    - This can be a sport, or some kind of physical activity.
    - Then make sure you put your absolute best effort into this activity to ensure highest intensity.

- If there isn't any specific cardio that you love, then the easiest way to increase **NEAT** without triggering hunger signals is take walks.
    - You could enjoy walks outside, or wherever it is you find enjoyable.
    - You could build the habit of taking the stairs rather than the elevator or escalator.
    - You could park the car further away from the location you're heading to, which allows more walking.
    - Conservatively estimating, on average (the average person, walking at a normal average pace), **3000-4000 steps = ~100 calories burnt**.
    - So a nice 1-hour walk consisting of 10,000 steps would burn approximately 300 calories. That's an excellent "deal" (movement for calories burnt), considering how easy it is, how little to none you've spent willpower on it, and how enjoyable it is.

Long story short, you don't want to do some mediocre cardio (especially if you hate it) that triggers all kinds of hunger signals, while in return it doesn't even burn that many calories. My recommendation is to either go extremely light or go crazy when it comes to burning calories through movement.

<u>Chapter 19</u>

SUMMARY OF THE DANGEROUS MYTHS

If you've read the book carefully up till now, it should've painted you a very clear picture of what you need to do to get to your dream physique. But because there's just so much noise out there, to make sure you stay on the right track and not start incorporating BS to slow down your progress, in this chapter, I'm going to give you a complete summary list of the common misconceptions you've heard or could hear in the near future.

1   "Artificial" or "chemicals" must be bad, "natural" must mean it's good.

This false assumption is known as "**natural fallacy**".

Artificial and natural are simply words to describe the methods they were obtained. The outcome of whether it's good for our bodies has nothing to do with these methods.

In fact, many artificial substances, such as medicine, are "good". Medicines can cure or treat illnesses. And many "natural" things can actually be harmful to us, such as cyanide, which is naturally occurring. A minuscule amount of cyanide is extremely poisonous for us.

And it's the same argument for "chemicals". Everything is, in fact, chemicals. The water we drink is H_2O, the simple sugar is $C_6H_{12}O_6$, and everything in our body is primarily made of carbon, hydrogen, oxygen, and nitrogen. They're ALL chemicals. Just because you never learned advanced chemistry and can't understand complex chemicals, doesn't make all of them instantly "bad" for you.

Some people, when referring to "chemicals", mean artificially synthesized chemicals. If that's the case, then the same argument about artificial versus natural above applies.

2   There is a secret trick to turn on a "fat-burning pathway", and you can then ignore calories, and you can eat any amount of food you want and never get fat.

We gain fat because of one reason - when there is an energy surplus in our body (through food). And magical "fat-burning pathways" that can be "cranked up" don't exist.

There's at least one BS like this every year. And none of them works because the property of fat loss is always this: the net energy balance in your body.

3   Fat gain is *caused* by hormonal or metabolic issues.

Fat gain could be WORSENED by hormonal or metabolic issues, but it's never directly CAUSED by them.

Just because your system is inefficient, doesn't mean that when there's no food (no energy), it could create body fat out of thin air. And just because your system is very efficient and healthy, doesn't mean that you can eat unlimited amounts of food (accumulate calorie surplus), and your body would just ignore them or discard them.

At the end of the day, there still needs to be an excess of energy for your body to store fat. If there's no excess energy, your body cannot gain fat, no matter what other issues it has.

4   A single type of food (fried food, meat, desserts, pizza, etc.) or nutrient (fats, carbs, saturated fats, sugar, etc.) causes fat gain.

Your body governs fat gain or loss at an "executive" level, decided depending on the overall net energy balance in the body. So no one single type of food or nutrient can directly cause fat gain. Only when there's an overall energy surplus, does the body begin to store the excess energy as body fat.

So if you ate all your food in the form of cookies, but somehow still manage to be in a calorie deficit, you'll lose fat regardless. And if you ate only fruits and veggies, but somehow were in a calorie surplus, you'll gain fat regardless.

5   A single type of food can boost your metabolism, significant enough to be relied on for fat loss.

Metabolism is simply total energy expenditure by your body's each and every function. More food does increase your energy expenditure because obviously you will need to digest it (and digesting costs energy). But digestion will NEVER cost more energy than the total energy of the food itself.

Imagine you ate 200 calories of cookies. Your body may spend a fraction of that calories to digest. And the remaining calories will still be stored as fat. But the digestion energy cost (thermic effect of food) will NEVER exceed 200 calories from the cookies.

It's like when you want to deposit $200 to your bank account, and the bank charges you a $2 processing fee. You still get to deposit $198. But imagine if the bank charged you $300 for the $200 you're depositing. Then the more you deposit, the less money you'd have. Would that make sense?

Your body is trying to survive by storing energy, not having less energy. So how can you expect a certain food to "boost metabolism" and burn fat by feeding it?

6   You should focus on "boosting metabolism" to lose fat.

Unfortunately, with the exception of physical activities, there are no ways of boosting metabolism in reliable ways to lose fat. The majority chunk of your overall net calories comes from food. So you need to focus on the calorie intake, not "boosting metabolism".

And even with physical activities, the amount of effort you put in to burn calories significant enough to create a calorie deficit is

NOT proportional. The "caloric return on cardio effort investment" is often very low, unless you absolutely love the activity. So if you put the majority of the emphasis on cardio purely for the sake of fat loss, you're making fat loss unnecessarily difficult.

7   A diet "works" because it has some fat-loss properties.

The only reason why your body stores fat is because there is an energy surplus in your body. So in order to lose fat, the only way is to be in an energy deficit. That's how it works.

So it doesn't matter if the diet is keto (improves insulin sensitivity), vegan (removes animal-related foods), intermittent fasting (tweaks meal timing), etc... if a diet works, it has to be because it somehow has put you in an energy deficit, and never because of some other magical reason. And if you ignored calories and ate without moderation, it doesn't matter what diet you're on, you won't lose fat.

8   You can spot-reduce fat (pick which body part you lose fat from).

Similar to what was mentioned earlier, the decision to burn fat or not is governed by a "higher level" executive system in your body, which means it's not localized. Exercising is, at best, for "adding" lean mass, NOT subtracting fat mass from a specific area.

9   Eating "healthy" automatically leads to fat loss.

When it comes to fat gain or loss, your body only cares about one thing: energy balance. Whether or not you label the food as "healthy" has nothing to do with it.

10   More cardio is always the answer to successfully getting lean.

As I've mentioned earlier in the book, even though cardio does burn calories, that doesn't always translate to a net energy deficit at the end, because of many factors, such as willpower, how much you actually enjoy that type of cardio, hormones and internal signals, and many more.

11   Being overweight or obesity is an illness, which is acquired outside of your control.

Being overweight or obese is the direct result of a prolonged accumulation of energy surplus. In simple terms, you ate too much! Therefore, obesity and being overweight isn't something you "catch", like a cold. It's predictable. So don't use this as an excuse, and take responsibility. Refer to misconception 3 above.

12   The "afterburn effect" from high-intensity interval training (HIIT) cardio is the "secret answer" to fat loss, and can be relied on for fat loss.

As I've already talked about earlier, it's about 10% of the total calories you burn from the HIIT session. Yeah... Not that much.

To put this into perspective, the average person burns about 300-400 calories per HIIT session. The afterburn effect is only about 30-40 calories for the entire next 48 hours. That's really it.

Don't chase the afterburn effect if you choose HIIT cardio. Don't do it because you think it's "good for fat loss". It's not particularly better than any other cardio. It's much more important to worry first about your diet and make sure you're in a calorie deficit. If you do ANY type of cardio, make sure you enjoy it. That means you're not using willpower to do it.

13   Eating at night makes you fat.

Same idea, only the overall energy balance, if being a surplus, can make you gain body fat. Meal timing itself doesn't directly cause weight change. Flip back to Chapter 10 for a more detailed answer.

Every once in a while, someone on the Internet will start some BS like "put cinnamon in water" or "cook with turmeric, the magical fat loss ingredient", etc. I hope that you'll smarten up after reading this book, and NEVER believe in any of these. The science behind how our body stores fat is extremely clear now. It ain't just an unsubstantiated hypothesis anymore. Trust me, there's no room for doubt, like "hey, maybe there's a secret way to lose fat that science hasn't found... maybe...".

Please, NO. Science is pretty clear already. So for your own good, kill the thought that there "could be" a new secret and not waste any time.

Chapter 20

FINAL WORDS

If you've read all the chapters in the book, and fully absorb what my book offers, I'm sure you'll have the following realizations:

1. You have a clear picture of what governs the appearance of your physique, and what you need to do.
2. Things aren't as difficult as you initially thought it'd be.
3. Things aren't as simple as you commonly hear it to be.

The reason why this book is called "The Dream Body Playbook", is because it can be the ONE book you will "play by" throughout your body transformation journey. The more you follow this book and the less distraction you listen to from elsewhere, the more successful you will be in terms of transforming into your dream physique. I've made the promise that it's the ONLY book you'll ever need to transform your body, and till this final chapter, it still holds true.

You may get a few thoughts as you go through your transformation process. Let me troubleshoot them here:

1   "I'm not getting the results that I want."

2   "It was working, but then the results seemed to have slowed down/plateaued/stopped altogether."

3   "It seems to be working, but how can I make this faster?"

To ALL those thoughts, here is my universal answer.

There are 2 possibilities:

1   You haven't given this journey enough time. Be patient.

YOU CAN'T MAKE THIS ANY FASTER (without sacrificing practicality). Trust me, I've already given you the fastest (and realistic) way. Using science, my own experience, and experience in coaching, I've concluded the fastest, most efficient lifestyle-friendly way for you. So kill that thought of seeking "faster" ways, and be patient. If you don't trust me, go ahead and waste your time doing other things. But don't blame me for not warning you that it'd be a waste of time, because you're going to wind up coming back to this anyway.

Or...

2   Re-read the book and relevant chapters. The answer is somewhere in there and you aren't really following it.

Or you might still be "free-styling" your own way, according to conventional wisdom and assumptions. The bottom line is, I've already laid out all the possibilities in the book, whether that's hitting a "plateau", or "feeling hungry", or "how much cardio you should be doing", or "how many calories you should be eating", or "when to eat more, when to eat less", etc etc. If you fully understood the book, you should know what to do.

So my recommendation is, after reading the book, during your body transformation journey, you're going to forget some things and that's okay. But GO BACK TO THE BOOK to find answers along the way. I promise you that 99% of the time, the answer is in there somewhere.

Now, you may be thinking, "this is too good to be true, why are you sharing so much valuable knowledge in just one book?"

Because I'm sick and tired of BS spewed by "professionals" in the fitness and health industry. It's rare to have people that are 1) not ignorant, 2) open-minded, 3) forward-science-thinking, and 4) selfless (providing services that are actually beneficial to people). Most "professionals" and businesses either A) don't have the actual scientifically-up-to-date knowledge, or B) have the knowledge, but are purposely selling other BS because the other BS is easier to sell to make money.

The fact of the matter is, in terms of body transformation, the most searched keyword phrase in Google is "how to lose belly fat", even though I think it should already be common sense by now that spot-reduction of body fat is not possible on any practical level. Yet many fitness and "health" businesses are still preying on the fact that most people don't understand all the underlying science, and they're selling you "fat-burning workouts" and "fat-burning superfoods", or "8-minute waist-tightening workouts". If you walk into a "healthy" food bar, what do you see? Smoothies and avocados, right?

So this BS ends here.

I hope you will put everything in this book to good use. I look forward to your body transformation. And give me a shout-out on my Instagram and other social media platforms if information in this book helped you transform. If I know that I did help you, it'll make me really happy as well.

Because this is what I live for.

Acknowledgements

First of all, I'd like to thank everyone who's supported me since day 1.

Special thanks to:

Ray Dong, for always believing in me since day 1; for supporting me through both words and actions; and for assuring me that I'm not that crazy for wanting to change the world (thankful that we share similar visions for the world).

David Lee, for being together with me on our self-development journey, always striving to be a better version of ourselves; for instigating this entire fitness pursuit, from a simple brother-like mutual promise of getting in better shape; and for always looking out for me like an older brother.

Umar Azhar, for always being there for me, and putting up with me; for being the best role model for me in morals and ethics; and for inspiring me to contribute good to society.

Ciara Wang, for believing in me since day 1, for your endless love and support, and for being the best learner and partner.

And all others, including but not limited to, Rachel S, Jerry Z, Ellie L, Jason A, Jeremy C, Tian Q...

Illustration Credits

Chapter 5

Chris Hemsworth, taken from the films, Thor

Eddie Peng Yu Yan, taken from Peng's Weibo page

Kendall Jenner, taken from Jenner's Instagram page @kendalljenner

Nana Un, taken from Un's Instagram page @nana.un

Chapter 6

Body fat visuals, parts of the image taken from the user, ZMNM, Imgur.com

Chapter 16

Recovery graphs, taken from cpsinmotion.com